T0348984

Praise for *Call the Nurse* and *Nurse, Come You Here!*

"Julia MacLeod shares unique and enchanting experiences as a nurse in rural Scotland. Her stories will ring true with every nurse—or anyone—who has ever cared for a family or a community, whether in Scotland or America. *Call the Nurse* is a delightful read."—LeAnn Thieman, author *Chicken Soup for the Nurse's Soul*

"Cozy and chatty . . . A lovely account of ordinary people thriving in an extraordinary landscape."—*Kirkus Reviews*

"The book feels like a letter from a friend who has an eye for travel writing. . . . With a nurse's no-nonsense manner, MacLeod relays tales of adventure, finding humor and humanity in her experiences. . . . For James Herriot fans, without the animals."—*Booklist*

"MacLeod proves to be an engaging narrative writer who uses humor and vernacular to her advantage. Should be of interest not only to medical professionals but to all readers who want to escape to a slower way of life."—*Library Journal*

"This lively and heartening memoir evokes both the hardships and the humour of island life."—*The Scotsman*

"This charming, bracing reminiscence of life on a remote Hebridean island captures a vanishing world filled with memorable stories and characters. . . . Mary J. MacLeod makes you care, moves you, amuses you, shocks you, teaches you: This is a surprising, satisfying memoir."—Floyd Skloot, author of *In the Shadow of Memory* and *The Wink of the Zenith: The Shaping of a Writer's Life*

"*Call the Midwife* gave [us] . . . the nursing profession in 1950s London. Now, a retired district nurse [gives us] the heartwarming and humorous—yet often shocking—events on a remote Scottish island."—*Sunday Post* (UK)

"A charming tale, packed full with reminiscences, rather in the manner of the recent hit TV series, *Call the Midwife*. . . . Her tales of joy, trouble, drama, and comedy are warm and humorous, telling of a bygone era."—*Westcountry Life*, *Western Morning News* (UK)

"Julia MacLeod has written a book which encapsulates Hebridean life during some decades past . . . with a sensitivity that reflects her nursing career."—Lady Claire Macdonald of Macdonald, from her foreword to *Call the Nurse*

"Not only about medical travails and emergencies, but also stories of friendship formed with steadfast people, children lost and found, farm animals that wander a little too far, and rumors of a ghostly apparition whispering a hidden secret. Extraordinary, heartwarming, and at times a little bit tragic, *Nurse, Come You Here!* captures the essence of a rugged, close-knit rural community."—*The Biography Shelf*

The
Country Nurse
Remembers

Also by Mary J. MacLeod

Call the Nurse
Nurse, Come You Here!

The
Country Nurse
Remembers

*True Stories of a Troubled
Childhood, War, and
Becoming a Nurse*

Mary J. MacLeod

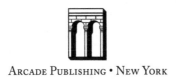

ARCADE PUBLISHING • NEW YORK

First North American Edition 2020

First published in 2015 by Luath Press Limited, Edinburgh, United Kingdom under the title *Hush! The Child is Present.*

Arcade Publishing books may be purchased in bulk at special discounts for sales promotion, corporate gifts, fund-raising, or educational purposes. Special editions can also be created to specifications. For details, contact the Special Sales Department, Arcade Publishing, 307 West 36th Street, 11th Floor, New York, NY 10018 or arcade@skyhorsepublishing.com.

Arcade Publishing® is a registered trademark of Skyhorse Publishing, Inc.®, a Delaware corporation.

Visit our website at www.arcadepub.com.

10 9 8 7 6 5 4 3 2 1

Library of Congress Cataloging-in-Publication Data

Names: MacLeod, Mary J., author.
Titles: The country nurse remembers : true stories of a troubled childhood, war, and becoming a nurse / Mary J. MacLeod.
Description: First North American Edition. | Published/Produced: New York : Arcade Publishing, 2020. | ©2015
Identifiers: LCCN 2019043261 (print) | ISBN: 9781950691296 (hardcover) | ISBN: 9781950691302 (ebook)
Subjects: MacLeod, Mary J.—Childhood and youth. | Nursing students England—Biography. | Stepdaughters—England—Biography. | World War, 1939–1945—Biography.
LC record available at https://lccn.loc.gov/2019043261

Cover design by Erin Seaward-Hiatt
Cover photographs: The author at the age of three with her mother; the author as a young student nurse

Printed in the United States of America

*This book is dedicated
to the memory of my mother,
whose love I knew for so short a time.
And to my baby sister, whom I did not know at all.*

CONTENTS

THE WAR YEARS

ACKNOWLEDGEMENTS

I thank all those members of my family and my friends who have encouraged me, especially my 'techno wizard', without whose help this book and others would probably not have been written.

INTRODUCTION

The story is of a confused, chaotic and repressive childhood lived in the West Country before, during and after the Second World War.

My childhood—in fact, my life as well—was very clearly defined by a 'Before' period and the 'After': before my mother died in 1937, when I was just five years old—these years are the lost time, the joyful time—and the events that followed after.

At her death, I was shunted from one relative to another, attending three different schools in as many months. My father was a man of his time, not expecting to look after a child himself, so he married again, only nine months after my mother's death, perhaps partly to have someone to look after me.

After my father's remarriage, my name was changed from my mother's choice of Mary to Julia. My father started to tell me that this new 'Mum', Mildred, was a better mother than my own would have been. Then my stepmother told me that my mother had not even wanted me. All these things made me an unhappy child, but I did not realise that I was unhappy. Things were just the way they were.

My experiences are set against a background of the Second World War. Evacuees came (and went); Father built an air-raid shelter; a plane crashed in the village; my stepmother's parents and cousin were bombed out in Bath and came to live with us for a while; German prisoners of war worked for my father for a while. There were sirens and air raids, and although the village escaped lightly we spent many nights in the shelter as bombs landed around us.

I gleaned what I could from playground talk, but my concept of events, local and global, was patchy, inaccurate. I was not allowed to listen to the wireless or read newspapers until late in the war, but those events that did enter my consciousness were to have a lasting effect on me and shape the way I thought for many years after.

I won a scholarship at eleven years old and tasted freedom from home, eventually choosing to study medicine and train as a nurse at Bristol Royal Infirmary. The hospital rules were severe but consistent, and I was 'growing up' all the time—learning about life as well as nursing.

I felt Mum's control gradually loosening, and I slowly began to have my own opinions and develop my own character, priorities and sympathies. I finished my three-year training, passed the final examinations and gained State Registration when I was twenty-one—officially an adult.

The 'Before' Time

The Child

'Hush! the child is present.'

Firmly, my grandmother admonished Grandfather. He had been sitting in his big leather armchair with his head in his hands. Crying, he had just murmured, 'I do grieve. Indeed, I do grieve!'

I was 'the child'—I knew that. And I knew why he was grieving.

Mummy

I was only five years old when my mother died. To me, she was the person who was always there, always loving, always ready to soothe or cuddle: able to find the lost doll, to locate the ice-cream van when we heard the 'ding-dong', to tuck me up in bed. I was safe, secure and fortunate—without knowing it. I took her presence and her love for granted. Then, suddenly, she was not there any more.

I had been taken to my grandparents' home nearby one day. They said, 'Mummy is not very well, but has gone away to hospital to get better and will soon be coming home again.' But she didn't come home again—ever.

My memories of that time and of my mother are fragmented, and I only pieced them together over a number of years. At the time I was not supposed to think about her—it was 'bad for me', she was 'best forgotten', I was told: I certainly did not dare ask about her or reminisce about 'when Mummy was alive'. It seemed that they all thought her death did not matter to me too much. 'The child does not appear to cry over her mother,' they said.

It mattered—oh yes, it mattered a great deal—but those were the days of the stiff upper lip, when children were to be seen and not heard, and we certainly didn't ask questions. In those days, a motherless child was a 'problem'.

The Country Nurse Remembers

Fathers rarely attempted the care of small children; some woman in the family was always found to do this. I knew nothing of the current attitudes, of course, but I could feel an atmosphere in the house, almost of embarrassment, that told me to remain silent: not to cry when among people and to hide away from all these things that I was deemed not to understand. I was not aware that I was miserable and lonely. Things were just the way they were.

I heard all the talk, or snippets of it: 'She does not understand,' 'She's a quiet child anyway,' 'She will soon forget—she is so young.' But I didn't forget—not for a minute.

Everyone talked about 'it' among themselves, but only once did anyone speak to me about Mummy's death, and that was immediately after she died (at least, I think it was). My father told me: 'Mummy has gone to see Jesus.'

At first, I wanted to ask why she could not come back when she had seen Jesus, and why had she not taken me with her to see Him? But I was a product of the old-fashioned attitudes, and had no proper religious teaching or understanding. I had a bluff, pre-occupied, unimaginative father who was doubtless in shock and grieving. So I kept all this worry to myself, and only by what I overheard was I able to understand that my mother had died. I knew what that meant. Death. And dying. I don't know *how* I knew. I think it was to do with a chicken that had been killed by a fox.

I remembered that the chicken had also 'gone to see Jesus'.

The Early Years

Mummy had been slim and rather elegant in the tube-like dresses of the 1930s. Naturally, as a small child, I did not think of her like this. Mummy was just Mummy: she smelled nice, had a soft voice and wore pretty dresses. I was an adult before I found a photo of her, and even now I have but three. One of them shows a smiling lady holding the hand of a small, rather thin little girl in a sun hat, walking along a seaside promenade. I must have been about four. Neither of us knew that this would be the last picture of us together: in less than a year, she had gone.

Another lovely memory of mine is her blowing up balloons for Christmas. I recall Mummy and my father putting up paper chains and then sitting by the fire with the balloons. I know that I sat watching them, and a warm feeling, even now, tells me that we were a happy threesome. My father had more 'puff', so he did the blowing, while my mother tied the balloons' necks. But she was not very good at it, and they kept zooming off across the room. I loved that!

I remember some words exactly.

'Why do you try to take the long end through the knot?' my father asked.

'I'll try the short end,' Mummy replied.

Pause.

'You've done the wrong one again,' he said.

'I did the short one, so now it is the long one's turn!'

Why should I remember such trivia when there must have been many other conversations that I overheard? Could it be that the atmosphere of love and joy etched this little piece of nonsense in my mind?

Then there was the doll episode. Again, I must have been about four, because I was going out of the front door by myself to play with some friends on the communal grassy area in front of the houses. I had in my arms a fairly large doll called Margaret. As I went down the steps, Mummy came running out, calling, 'Don't take your dolly—those boys might get her again!' By which I gather 'those boys' had caused trouble with Margaret before.

I must have been an adventurous child. We moved house soon after this, and there were some derelict buildings on the opposite side of a wide, shallow stream which ran in front of our house now. I was warned sternly by Father not to go there, as they were unsafe, and, so far as I remember, I did not go into these buildings but spent much time standing beside the stream looking at them. Occupied in this way one day, I was startled by an old man emerging from one of them and shouting at (or to) me. I was terrified, and, in my hurry to escape, I fell into the stream.

I was in no danger: the stream was so shallow, and this 'ogre' of a man was kindness itself, pulling me out, establishing, with difficulty, where I lived and returning me to my mother. She was not at all cross but wrapped me up, cuddled me to get me warm, and then made the old tramp a cup of tea. Father, however, was cross when he came home, but, as always, Mummy smoothed things over by saying, 'She didn't go into those houses. She was only looking at them.' I remember my father's 'Hmm.'

My next two adventures must have happened in the few months before her death. I had a tricycle and was persuaded to go out with some friends who were also the proud owners of similar small trikes. Near our home some new houses were to be built, and the roads had been laid out and partially surfaced ready for work to begin. Since they were totally free of traffic and ran down the side of a hill, they were considered by my friends (all of whom were a good three or four years my senior) to be most suitable for a good 'whizz'. And they were!

I began to whizz with the rest, but the trike was new, and, unfortunately, I had not mastered the use of the brakes. Faster and faster I went! I remember the shouts of encouragement behind me. We were all totally oblivious to the dangers. The road ended in a T-junction, and I failed to negotiate the corner and was unable to stop. I careered across the road and hit the newly installed curb with my head.

I woke sitting on a stool in the workmen's hut, with a grubby but kindly man sponging the warm sticky stuff that was pouring from a cut on my forehead. At that moment, my father arrived, having been fetched by the other children. Pressing his handkerchief to my head, he wrapped me in something and carried me to the car. Holding the mangled tricycle out of the open driver's window with his right hand—I remember that so vividly—he drove me home to a distraught mother who was being regaled by the children's tale of accident and blood—much embellished, I believe. Sometime later, I recall Father saying to my mother, 'I want to give those chaps something for their kindness.' I don't remember what they received.

While still with plasters all over my face, I went to call on a little friend. On her doorstep was her very old spaniel, sleeping soundly. I was very fond of dogs, so I bent to pat him, startling the old dog, which had not heard my approach. Frightened, he turned quickly and bit instinctively. My already battered face received several additional bites, as did my neck. For some reason, instead of knocking on the door, I ran all the way home, once more with blood pouring from me and terrifying my poor mother. But I know that I received love and comfort. Perhaps I had been foolish, but it was an accident and that was the end of the matter.

I think it was with the same little friend that I shared my next adventure. I believe her name was Audrey, and I remember her as being small and always dressed in blue. She was slightly younger than I was, and therefore I was considered to be the ringleader in our games or escapades.

Near 'the house with the stream in front', as I always thought of it, there was a little park with flowers and swings. One afternoon we went there and spent a long time on the swings. We tried to outdo each other to see how high we could go before the ropes bent and jerked. I seem to remember that we went very high!

These days, parents would be unlikely to allow five-year-olds to go to a park, even a nearby one, unaccompanied. But life was safer for children then, and we were free to make our own fun.

At the park, there was an old man who swept up and kept an eye on the children's area. We spent a long time chatting to him from the swings. He must have been a patient old fellow because he kept saying that he would have to shut the gates, and we kept saying, 'Just one more swing.' We were the only ones left there and I remember that the sun had gone in, but as children we had no idea of time. The old man did not tell us to go but kept asking if our mummies would be worried about us. With great confidence, we assured him that we were allowed in the park. I don't suppose he knew what to do with us.

Suddenly, there was a commotion at the gate, and Daddy and Audrey's father came striding towards us. They stopped to speak to the man, who smiled and nodded towards us. We got off the swings and ran to the two daddies—with our usual grins, no doubt.

We were amazed when we saw their faces. I think they were cross and relieved at the same time. We had apparently been out for hours and had forgotten to tell our mothers where we were going. And it was not that the sun had just gone in . . . No, it was getting dark!

We were scooped up and given a good talking to, plenty of hugs and a piggy back home. Poor Mummy greeted me with tears of relief, as she held me tightly. I couldn't understand this at all. We had been fine, I reasoned.

I remember being made to sit down and listen to Daddy telling me why they were worried. There was a long, deep brass fender in front of our fire, and two square leather-topped wooden boxes, like small ottomans, were attached at each end to form seats. One held old newspapers and one contained sticks, both for lighting the fire. I used to like sitting on these, and I can almost smell the brown leather as I remember my mother holding my hand that night as I sat on a box as Daddy talked.

All these years later, I can still feel the warmth of my mother's love, known for just those few years, not even understood, but perhaps more precious because it all ended so soon.

Grandparents and Aunts

There were other members of both my parents' extended families who lived fairly near us and so were part of my early life. When at my father's parents' home at 'Meadow View', I had to be 'grown-up' even at the age of four. These grandparents seemed very, very old to me, probably because they both suffered ill health in different ways.

Grandma had been totally blind from the age of about thirty. As a very small child, I understood that this meant she could see nothing at all, so I wondered how she knew when I came into the room or where in the room I happened to be. I was sure that she had a magic way of knowing when I was there and where things were kept, like Grandpa's slippers or the ornaments on the side tables. Much later I learned that her hearing had become more acute as her blindness progressed and she had developed the ability to interpret little sounds, such as footsteps. She could judge the rough weight of a person by the noise that the feet made on the floor, so she knew if it was a child or an adult. She also had a phenomenal memory for the way in which everything was arranged in the house. Woe betide anyone who moved anything without warning her! It must have happened, though, because I remember her poor wrinkled face always had bruises where she had bumped into a half-opened door or fallen over a chair carelessly left protruding from the table.

She had a dog called Flossie, a gentle, fluffy creature, who happened to be blind too. Flossie always moved out of Grandma's way when she heard her feet coming but would stubbornly remain where she had decided to lie if anyone else tried to pass. She seemed to understand that we could see her, while Grandma could not. 'Doggie magic', I believed. I remember asking one day if we were 'going to see Flossie' and having to be reminded that we were going to see Grandma and Grandpa too! I loved Grandma and Flossie in about equal amounts, I think.

I was afraid of Grandpa. As a result of a stroke, his left hand had set in a claw-like shape, and he had no real appreciation of the strength that still remained in it. He would play at 'rough and tumble' with my cousins and me and had no idea that he was hurting us by squeezing, prodding or pulling us. We had all been told that Grandpa 'had a bad hand' and we must not complain if he hurt us because 'he can't help it'. We did as we were told (of course) but often tried to slink away so that he should not see the tears. I can remember the terror I felt one day when he held me down for so long that I thought I was going to scream. That would not have done at all!

Under his rather rough exterior, however, he must have been something of a gentleman because one day, to our enormous relief, he decided that we were getting to be 'young ladies' (at five or six years old) and it was not 'seemly' to play-fight anymore.

When I look back on these times at my grandparents', it is often without the warm feeling that trickled down through those years when my mother was alive; I can't hear a voice in my head that could have been hers. This makes me think these years must belong to the 'after' time. But, then again, it was perhaps just that her quiet presence was somehow overwhelmed by my father's large family of a brother, a sister, nephews, nieces and, it seemed, an endless parade of aunts, all of whom seemed to look alike to me.

Auntie Jinny

There was one aunt who stood out from the rest: Auntie Jinny. She was not part of the great gaggle of aunts in my father's family but rather my mother's aunt, so in fact she was a great aunt to me. She was a tiny lady who had lost her husband in the Great War. She spoke of this long-dead, much-loved heroic man with great reverence.

She always referred to the 'Great' War, so I thought it was something splendid, imagining shining armour and glossy horses. It was only after school history lessons that I realised she meant the First World War. (The Second World War was a few years ahead then, and so the Great War was still thought of as the war to end all wars.)

She lived in a tiny cottage in a little town in the Cotswolds, and we used to go to stay with her quite often when my mother was still alive. My father did many odd jobs for her about the cottage while I 'helped' to dig the garden. Mummy would rattle about in the stark kitchen making all manner of nourishing foods for Auntie, being convinced that she did not eat properly because she lived alone. The kitchen was more of a scullery because the actual cooking was done on a huge old range which stretched the length of the living room and was faithfully black-leaded daily. The big china sink in the kitchen was very low down, supported on two little brick walls, while a board placed across one end of the room held back the coal heap. I remember a lot of talk about the dust from the coal getting into the food, but we just washed the dust off the plates before we used them. Daddy said it was 'clean dirt'.

The front door led straight into the living room from the pavement. In order to reduce draughts and add a little privacy from passers-by when the door was open, a huge settle was placed inside the doorway to hide the room. Looking back now, I believe it had been a church box-pew before being demoted to Auntie's cottage. In front of the fire (the open part of the range) was a rag-rug that I remember Auntie once repairing with some old stockings. I was allowed to cut the thick material into small pieces for her to hook into the holes in the ancient rug. A comfortable old settee faced the fire, while a sort of chaise longue (Auntie did not call it that—it was the 'couch') was placed against the wall under the window. I used to stand on this and watch the people walking past. Somewhere in the room there was a square, highly polished dining table with a huge china 'something' in the middle. The room must have been smaller than I remember and probably very cluttered, but I loved that room!

There was no bathroom in the cottage, and I remember being washed in front of the fire and my clothes warmed on the fender. The lavatory was in a little brick building outside the back door. It was very cold in the winter, but I liked the picture of Jesus that hung on the wall.

Many more pictures of a golden-haired Jesus, with a shining halo, adorned the rest of the cottage, as did images of a stately St. Francis. I liked the animals and birds that always surrounded him. Another picture showed God sitting on a cloud, and I know I used to feel uneasy sometimes when it rained because I would worry that God would get very wet. But where did he sit when there were no clouds? That was another worry. I was intrigued by a particular picture showing Jesus knocking at a door overgrown with weeds. Much, much later I learned that this was a print of the famous Holman Hunt painting. I think Auntie's interpretation of these pictures was about the nearest I got to any understanding of what it was all about because my father prided himself on being an agnostic. None of this made sense to a four- or five-year-old, but I loved Auntie, I loved the pictures and I was happy in her cottage, so I associated God and Jesus with a warm, comfortable feeling.

Interspersed among the religious pictures were so many photographs of family members that it was difficult to see the flowered wallpaper. One day my father asked Auntie Jinny to name one or two of them. Her reply caused a lot of laughter: 'I can't remember their names,' she said, 'because several have been dead for years.' But the photos were still there the next time we visited her.

The staircase opened from a kind of cupboard beside the range. It had a latch door. If my father stood on the floor at the bottom of the stairs, he could place his hand on the floor of the tiny landing: the ceilings were so low and the stairs so steep.

There were only two bedrooms, both with steeply sloping ceilings. Mummy and Daddy slept in the front and larger room, which was kept aired for guests, while I slept in the double bed, on a feather mattress, with Auntie Jinny in the smaller room at the back. I was on the inside, under the slope of the ceiling. If I sat up without thinking, I banged my head; it was so low.

The back gardens of the row of cottages were all joined together; there were no fences between them. There were narrow paths running down the gardens and across them, made from years and years of ashes from the fires, and in the squares of ground all the neighbours grew cabbages, peas, carrots and all manner of vegetables and soft fruit and shared the produce among them. I loved to run up and down and across these paths, pretending that they were roads. At the bottom of the gardens was a brook with tadpoles and frogs and sometimes a water vole.

I loved it! All of it: Auntie, her cottage, staying there with Mummy and Daddy, the laughter and the quiet chats about 'dear Frank' and about God. Auntie was the only person in the family who spoke of such things (and certainly the only one who spoke about my 'dear mother' after her death). She loved Mummy and me; in fact, she seemed to love everyone. She had no children, and, although she would have loved to have had a child, she said, 'If God had wanted me to have children, He would have *given* me children.' Those were the days when one accepted such things, rather than moving heaven and earth to change them.

Auntie Jinny was the link between the time 'before Mummy died' and the time 'after Mummy died', which was how I thought of my life. Even then, when that life was not very good, we went to see her. I cherished those times! They were like an oasis in an otherwise bleak world because instinctively I knew that she loved me. She was the only person who spoilt me and spent time with me when my mother was no longer there.

She talked about my mother in a natural way: with sadness, but not in the hushed, embarrassed way that others did, if they said anything at all. Later still, when even the mention of my mother became taboo, she still spoke of her and would not be silenced.

Great Aunt Louisa and Grandmother

There was another aunt on my mother's side: a very different lady from Auntie Jinny. She was Great Aunt Louisa and she suited her name. I was always overawed when we went to tea in her elegant flat, which had been left to her by her employers. She had been a lady's maid to an aristocrat in Cheltenham and had frequently attended her at the Royal Court, absorbing much of that way of life. She had acquired a very precise way of speaking, which gave her an autocratic bearing.

When we arrived, the door would be opened by the 'daily' (who never seemed to have a name), and we would be shown in to the drawing room, a long, rather cold room with huge windows. After curtsying slightly, while being greeted, I was expected to answer questions about every aspect of my young life. Her opinions would then be offered about any shortcomings, as she saw them, in my upbringing and general behaviour. After that the 'daily' would bring in tea in small cups, tiny cucumber sandwiches and dainty cakes. I would be given a glass of milk because it was not socially correct for small children to drink tea, we were told. Oddly, I was not afraid of her, as one might have expected. I think I was fascinated by this glimpse into a different world.

After my mother's death, Great Aunt Louisa would not entertain my father, so I did not see her again. When she died, however, she left me £100, which was a lot of money in 1950!

Great Aunt Louisa was my maternal grandmother's sister. Grandmother was a stickler for social niceties in much the same way as Great Aunt Louisa, and, although kind and careful of my emotional well-being ('Hush! The child is present'), she seemed remote, reserved and unapproachable. I must have spent much time with those grandparents before my mother's death, but I do not remember any hugs, just a peck on the cheek on arrival and another when I left.

Grandfather was a bank manager, which was considered to be a very good job in those days, and he always seemed to be going out of the front door in a pinstripe suit with a bowler hat, carrying a rolled umbrella and a briefcase, or coming in looking exactly the same.

I never saw Grandfather open the big briefcase, but one day I was bold enough to ask him what was in it. He humphed a bit, saying in an irritated way, 'Papers, child, papers!' I was no wiser but dared not ask again.

Their house smelled of furniture polish and had soft carpets. There was a formal dining room, a parlour and a great big kitchen, where I had my meals.

Crib

I loved Meadow View, Grandma's and Grandpa's house, better than Grandmother's house, because it was not so precise and there were animals there: Flossie and Crib, and the three big shire horses.

Crib was a big bull terrier, an outside dog, a working dog. The waste-water treatment plant, which we called the Works, and the horses' stables were infested with rats and mice, so Grandpa had bought Crib and trained him to eliminate them.

I loved Crib in a different way from the fluffy, cuddly Flossie, who was so gentle. Crib was lively, cunning and deadly to rats, cats and even other dogs (other than Flossie, whom he adored), but he was the champion protector of small children such as me and my cousins. We would put him on a rope and march him round the garden, supposedly taking him for a walk. Compared with his free and busy life, this must have been quite boring, but he happily trotted with us, tail wagging. He would join in our hide-and-seek, crouching behind a bush or a building until someone would find us, and he would leap about in ecstasy, having no idea what all the fuss was about but delighted to be part of our game.

The Country Nurse Remembers

One weekend, when Daddy and Mummy and I were staying at Meadow View, two small friends joined my cousin Ellen and me for a game of hide-and-seek in the garden—but this time the grown-ups had to find us. They gave us a good long time to get hidden and then they began the search. After some time they must have started to worry, as I could hear Daddy saying, 'What have they got up to now?' then, 'They have been gone too long.'

We were trying not to giggle when we heard him say, 'I think that dog knows something. Look at him, sitting there in the doorway of his kennel. He looks far too pleased with himself.' But we could contain ourselves no longer and pushed our way out of the huge kennel past Crib, who had been doing a grand job of hiding us by filling the doorway with his huge bulk. He joined our victory dance with barks and leaps, and the event joined all the other stories that grew around Crib.

When he was not working, he would often be chained to the kennel, which was placed beside the garden path. It must have been there for years because all sorts of grass and weeds were growing around it, so that it looked partially buried. I used to annoy Grandpa by saying that Crib would be cold.

'He's a tough outside dog and he's got a warm straw bed in there. He's fine!' he'd say.

He certainly seemed fine. He was a big, muscular dog, healthy and alert. One day he was chained outside the kennel as usual, when a mouse ran past his nose on its way up the garden path. In no time, Crib was after it, dragging the enormous kennel and assorted plants and turf with him. He must have had great strength to pull it virtually out of the ground. And he caught the mouse!

Grandpa had a hazy photo of Crib, sitting against the house wall at about nine a.m. one day, looking extremely smug. Tied across the wall behind him were some pieces of string holding the remains of ten rats and several mice. He had caught and killed all these before breakfast.

The men used to take Crib to the Works early in the morning and just let him loose in the stables and other buildings. They would troop back for a full breakfast at about nine a.m., and when Crib saw the preparations for the return home (perhaps he was to have his breakfast, too) he would gather the dead rats by their tails and jauntily trot back with them. I'm not sure what Grandma thought of this: she would have smelled them even though she could not see them.

These were good times.

Fun, Floods and Peter the Pup

I know that I must have forgotten many, many things that happened in the 'before time'—that is, before my mother died—because I was so young. But I certainly have not forgotten the celebrations in May 1937 for the Coronation of King George VI. Mummy and Daddy took me to Victoria Park in Bath to see the fireworks and hear the bands playing. I remember lots of people laughing and shouting and the darkness being split by swooshing rockets. We walked along a wide path, watching and listening to all the fun. I had never seen so many people, and Mummy and Daddy held my hands very tightly as I skipped excitedly. I felt quite grown-up because I was out in the dark. I was told that we had a new king, which would not have meant much to me, but none of that mattered—it was all such fun. I remember the bright lights shining on the underside of the leaves on the trees that lined the road. I thought that fairyland must be like this. Then Daddy bought some sparklers from a stall, lit one and handed it to me, telling me to hold it well away from my face. All was well for a while, but as it began to burn down I became frightened and tried to flick it away. It stuck to my woolly glove and flicked straight into my face. I recall being worried that this would mean that we would have to go home. I wasn't bothered about the stinging sensation on my cheek. It could not have been very bad because after the inevitable fuss and an inspection of my face, Daddy picked me up so that I could see better and we stayed on until Mummy became tired.

We must have been living in Bath at that stage because a few days later, I think, when we went to visit Grandma and Grandpa and Flossie at Meadow View, we had to go in the car. It would have been about five miles. As we began to go down the lane bordering the river, we had quite a shock. It was flooded! There were some gnarled old willow trees growing on the river bank beside the lane and these seemed to me to be floating, the water was so high.

Daddy got out and walked to where the lane disappeared into the water. He returned, saying that it was not too deep and we would manage it. To me, peering from the back window as we drove slowly through the water, it was all very exciting—almost as good as the Coronation. But it was over too soon. When we reached the dry part of the lane, we seemed to be hopping along in a series of leaps and jumps, but that, too, was fun. Much later I was told that Daddy was drying the brakes. We must have done the same thing on our return, or perhaps the water had retreated, as I have no memory of it at all.

Daddy called his car 'Tin Lizzy'. It was an Austin 7, black with nice-smelling leather upholstery. I loved the smell of Tin Lizzy—and even liked the smell of the petrol. (Petrol was less than an 'old' shilling a gallon at the time, just fivepence!) We had lots of outings in Tin Lizzy in the 'before' time—and in the 'just after' time.

My father must have sold her soon after my mother died because the next car was a blue Ford, which we called 'Bluebird'.

While we still had Tin Lizzy, we used to take Grandma out for rides. I used to wonder why she liked this because she couldn't see anything. I think she just liked the company. One day we took her with us for a picnic. We ate jam sandwiches and had tea out of a thermos. Suddenly, Grandma cried out and Mummy and Daddy rushed to her. A wasp, which had landed on the jam in her sandwich, had stung her face. Daddy quickly sucked the poison out, spitting it onto the ground while Mummy held Grandma's hand. Whether we had to go home or how bad Grandma was, I don't recall, but I was very impressed with Daddy's quick action in sucking out the poison. Even today, this is still the quickest way to relieve the pain of a wasp or bee sting.

There are many other stories surrounding Tin Lizzy, but whether I actually recall these or whether others have told me, I don't know. Sometimes people can tell such vivid tales that you could easily think that you remember the incident yourself.

Peter the Pup, however, was real enough. I can't picture where we were living at the time—in the house by the stream or the house with the grass in front—and I do not even remember Daddy actually bringing Peter the Pup home. He was just there one day. A small, slim short-haired mongrel, I loved him as soon as I saw him.

I once got cross when he knocked down my carefully built tower of bricks, but I was allowed to play with them on the table, and Peter the Pup was back in favour.

We used to chase about outside, and up and down the stairs and in and out of the table legs. But we never took him with us when we went to see Grandma and Grandpa! 'You don't want to let Crib see him,' Daddy said. 'He might think he is a rat!' Crib's great prowess with rats and his bad reputation with cats might have extended to small dogs, it seemed.

Peter the Pup had a bad habit of wandering off, and he wasted a lot of Daddy's time, trying to locate him. Some local lads offered to help on several occasions, and Daddy gave them sixpence every time.

One day I heard Daddy say, 'I think those boys are enticing that dog away so as to get sixpence for bringing him back. I'll have to see these scallywags.' 'Scallywag' was a favourite word of Daddy's.

Peter the Pup did not go missing as often after that.

We often took Peter the Pup on picnics with us, when we'd all sit on the ground on rugs. One hot day, Uncle Jake and Auntie Aggie and their four children were with us. They had one car, and Daddy took Grandma and Grandpa, Mummy and me.

We pulled off the road into the shade of a sort of wood with big open spaces in a place called Burrington Combe. There was some joking because one of my cousins was picking some flowers and the grown-ups pretended that a policeman would come and tell him off. (Actually, the picking of wild flowers was allowed at that time.)

At that moment, a policeman did appear, and, after a bit of banter, he 'booked' (Daddy's word) Daddy and Uncle Jake for parking more than fifteen yards from the highway. I had never heard the road called 'the highway' before. It made it sound very grand, but it was only a lane. I was a bit scared, thinking that they would be sent to prison, but they all had a laugh with 'that copper', telling him about the flower-picking joke.

About a week later, they were both fined, and Daddy said that it was very unfair as it was the first time that he had ever been 'had up'. I can still remember the two cars, in the clearing with the dappled sunlight and lots of moss and green logs. We jumped off these and ran about playing hide-and-seek while the grown-ups did boring things like smoking and chatting.

There is a warm feeling as I remember that day, partly because my two girl cousins were still children in the way that I was— wearing much the same type of clothes as I did, so I felt the same as them. When we were a few years older, after my mother's death and things were very different, I felt silly and embarrassed when I was with them, as they were allowed to wear more grown-up clothes but I was still made to wear childish dresses, lace-up shoes and knickers with elastic round the legs. My hair was kept very short and straight, while they grew theirs and had plaits or loose curls.

But my cousins had never had a dog and I had Peter the Pup! I loved that dog, but I have no idea what happened to him. Like so much in that time after Mummy died, no one was there to explain it to me. He was just not there anymore.

The Shire Horses and Crib—Again

Before mummy died, and afterwards, when I lived at Meadow View, I was able to see quite a lot of the horses. They were three big Shires: Punch, Charlie and Old Bob.

Old Bob was a tall, black horse who was getting very old and no longer worked. He had been 'retired', said Daddy, and just stood about and munched grass. He was always ready to come to the fence for a carrot. Daddy used to lift me up to give this to him, as he was so tall.

Punch and Charlie were brown and not quite so tall but had very big, lovely hairy feet. They still had to work. They made hay, they ploughed, they dragged various things about the Works and generally farmed the land that formed part of the whole waste-water treatment plant area. They were placid and friendly. They had a sort of stable for the cold weather and several fields for the summer.

Before my mother died, Grandpa or Daddy used to take me along to the blacksmith. There was no farrier, apparently (although I would not have known what one was), so the blacksmith did the shoeing. This was usually the way for working horses in the countryside in those days: farriers were mostly

28

used for racehorses or by rich people who rode horses about for fun.

The blacksmith lived in the village on the hill, on the opposite side of the river, so there was a special ferry to take the horses across the water. It was a big, old flat-bottomed, almost square, sort of boat—almost like a floating bridge. It was made of old planks that had the scuff marks of generations of horses' hooves. One end could be let down to form a ramp from the bank for the horses to board. There was no engine, and one of the chaps usually poled it across a shallow part of the river and then walked the horse up through the fields to the forge. Daddy would drive us up there by road. It was a very long way round, as we had to go to the next village before there was a bridge, or all the way into Bath in the other direction. This is why there was a horse ferry.

I loved the forge. It was always warm, with its fire and the bellows. Then there were all the things that the blacksmith made apart from horseshoes, such as gates and fancy things for rich people's gardens. He was a big man with a very bushy black beard, a red face and a loud, gurgling laugh. He always gave me a sweet from the blackest hands that I ever saw, but I was told that they were not really dirty: it was just the soot from the fire. There was a sort of stone seat against the wall, and I would be told to sit there and watch.

The horse, perhaps Punch, would be led in. Mr. Blacksmith would talk to him and pat his neck and then lift his feet one at a time, take off the old shoes and scrape the hooves. 'Paring the hooves', I was told. Then the blacksmith would work the bellows with one foot, while making the new shoe, or altering the old one. The shoe would be red hot—I could feel the heat from my seat by the wall—and then there would be much hissing and steam (or perhaps it was smoke), and the shoe would be placed against the hoof that Punch so quietly offered. I took a lot of convincing that the hot shoe did not hurt him as it was pressed onto his hoof. Then the nails, each one held in the blacksmith's mouth, were banged in. Again, I winced with every bang until I was shown that the horse did not feel any pain because the hoof was 'dead' just like my fingernails.

During all this, there was much grown-up talk about the weather, something called 'the corporation' and something else called 'income tax'. I don't know why I remember little things like that, for I had no idea what it was all about: I just sat and watched and was happy. I didn't know that I should have treasured those times—as they would stop all too soon.

When the shoeing was done, Daddy and I would go into the house for a cup of tea with Mrs. Blacksmith while 'the chap' took Punch back across the fields to the horse ferry and across the river in his new shoes.

Just as my days of visiting the blacksmith stopped, so too did those of the heavy horse. Thankfully, we were behind the times and carried on using our horses for years, because when the war came and people had problems getting fuel for tractors and lorries, many people wished that they had kept their animals.

Old Bob, however, must have reached the end of his life at about the beginning of the war. Grandpa and Daddy decided that it was best to have him put to sleep, and the vet was sent for with his gun. I remember Daddy had tears in his eyes as he told me that the old fellow had gone. I was very sad too and cried at the thought that I would not see Old Bob again.

Punch and Charlie lived into the time of the war and beyond, though I do not remember what happened to them (I had probably left home by the time their end came).

So the shoeing at the blacksmith went on for some years, but later on I was not allowed to go to the forge. Why? Like so much else, I don't know.

The Country Nurse Remembers

I missed the times with Daddy, and I missed Punch and Charlie.

* * *

I think Crib, however, was my favourite animal. But how he hated cats! To him, they were probably just another sort of rat or rabbit, and everyone praised him for catching those. And because of where we lived—with few neighbours and surrounded by fields with haystacks (and haystacks attract mice and cats love to catch mice . . .)—there were quite a few semi-feral cats around, in addition to some pet cats belonging to a nearby farm.

While Mummy was still with us and we stayed at Meadow View, I would sometimes wake early to hear Daddy in the garden as he dug yet another grave to bury someone's cat before they missed it. I know now that none of these cats were real pets, but I worried then in case someone was sad. But Daddy was protecting Crib from irate farmers, I think.

There was one story about Crib that was told for years. Daddy smoked in those days and used to walk up the lane with Crib to have a last smoke before bedtime. One night, a small black dog appeared from our neighbour's wooden bungalow (they didn't have a dog—perhaps someone was visiting with this Scottie). Crib saw him and gave chase. He caught him in no time and started to bite him round the neck. Daddy said 'he meant business'. There was a lot of snarling and growling, he said, and then Crib would not let go. Daddy hauled him back, even kicked him—he did everything to try to separate the two fighting dogs.

'The little 'un didn't stand a chance,' said Daddy.

Eventually, he caught them both by the scruff of their necks and, with his big, strong arms, swung them round and round, releasing them when they were high enough to sail over the hedge into the field with the haystacks.

'Crib is bound to let go as they land,' he thought.

But Crib did not let go. Daddy was amazed to hear the snarling continue on the other side of the hedge. He pushed his way through and again attempted to part them by getting between them—a dangerous thing to do! He was bitten and shouted in pain. Immediately, Crib let the small dog go and skulked on his tummy towards Daddy because he thought he had bitten his master. Luckily, it was the other dog that had bitten, and the wound was not as deep as it would have been had Crib's big teeth done the damage. The little dog ran off, a bit bloodied but not badly hurt.

Daddy wore a large bandage for several days, and Crib was tied up at the kennel until the little dog and his owners left. I used to love hearing this story, imagining Daddy swinging the two dogs round and round at shoulder height and then letting them sail over the hedge.

Understanding

All these good times changed on the day that my father told me of my mother's death.

We were at the home of my grandmother and grandfather Radford, Mummy's parents. My father took me into the hallway (I think there were people in the parlour) and told me while we sat on the plush red-carpeted stairs. I already knew that something was wrong because Grandmother had red eyes and Grandfather had suddenly seemed to shrink. Father held me tightly after he told me about Mummy 'going to see Jesus'. It was lovely to have him cuddling me, but I was crying and I wanted to blow my nose, so I had to wriggle away to get my hankie. I was full of questions: 'Is she coming back?', 'Can we go to meet her?', 'Why?', 'How long?' . . . But because I voiced none of these my father thought that I understood. He went back to the adults, and Grandmother called me into the kitchen to have my tea. So far as they were concerned, I had been told and that was that.

In the kitchen, another person whom I called Aunt but who was not a 'real' aunt put bread and butter before me, and as she stroked my hair she started to cry. She talked to me, but I wished she wouldn't. Later I learned that she was totally deaf, which explains why she spoke with such a loud voice and why it was often hard for me to understand her. I thought she was kind, but I always worried in case I seemed rude. On this occasion, Grandmother came in and instructed her: 'Dry your eyes and pull yourself together.'

My aunt—I think her name was Daphne—immediately ran from the room and left me with Grandmother. She talked to me about my tea, my toys and so on in her clear, kind but rather clipped tones. The rest of the day, in fact the next few days, was a blur. I just remember missing Mummy.

I gradually came to realise that she was dead, dead, dead.

The blur must have lasted through the funeral, but no one told me that there was one. I just stayed with Grandmother, played with my dolls and ate my food, and was probably taken for walks in the park.

Then suddenly I became a pupil at a 'dame school' on the outskirts of Bath. It was not far from Grandmother's house, so she took me there each day. The school was in a big Victorian house and was run by two elderly ladies. Or perhaps they were only 30 or so; they just seemed old to me. It was rather posh, so I think it was Grandmother's choice, and I always felt that Daddy did not really approve of the school. Perhaps his in-laws were paying for it. I don't remember anything specific but just a certain grim look on his face on the occasions that he delivered or collected me.

I do remember being rather unhappy at first, as I started there so soon after losing my mother, but I made friends with two sisters, who must have been twins, who mothered me. There were only about six little girls, all aged within a few years of my five years old, but I remember the two sisters were eight. They had just obtained something called a scholarship to another school and seemed very grand and grown-up to me. I was comforted by their friendship.

Then one day Daddy came to the school during dinner time and went into the study with the two ladies. When they all emerged, I was told to pick up my pencils and drawing books and say goodbye because I was going to go to a different school. The ladies were rather stiff with Daddy but were kind to me and said that they hoped I would like my new school. These days a child would ask questions, I'm sure; make objections, possibly indulge in tears or tantrums and undoubtedly explanations would follow. But I did nothing, asked nothing and possibly felt nothing. I was just a child being told what was to happen, so I just collected my things and followed my father to the car. I remember an empty feeling as I waved to the ladies, but I just did what was expected of me. I was there to be taken or sent wherever it was deemed right.

When I look back I think surely I must have asked why I had to go to another school. But no! I just climbed dumbly into the car.

Another shock awaited me at Grandmother's house.

In the hall was a little case with my heavy coat draped over it and, beside it, a basket with my dolls and books. Grandmother bustled me into the kitchen for milk and biscuits while my father put my case and toys into the car. Only then was I told what had been decided for me.

'You are going to live with Auntie Doris, now.'

I would have nodded and accepted the news, even though I hardly knew Auntie Doris. She was Mummy's sister—I had been a bridesmaid at her wedding to Uncle John only a few months earlier. I had worn a yellow dress and a floral headband and had carried a little silk purse that matched the dress. I still have the tinted photograph. I had been so proud and happy then, and my aunt and uncle had seemed nice. But we hardly ever saw them now, as they lived in Bristol.

Bristol and Bath seem very close these days, but the road from one to the other was narrow and winding then, and the towns themselves were much smaller, with large stretches of countryside in between, so the distances seemed greater. And now, suddenly, I was going to live with virtual strangers in a different town.

'Are you going to live there too, Daddy?' I wanted to know.

'No, I've got to go to work. And I've got to finish the bungalow.'

Daddy was building a bungalow beside the river in the village where Grandma and Grandpa lived. He had been planning for us to live in it—it was nearly finished—but Mummy had died before we could move in. Looking back over the years, I can see how that must have been an added blow to my father: to be building, in his spare time, a home for his wife and family, and having that wife die before he could take her there. Typically, he said little, but I wonder what his thoughts were later, when we did eventually move in.

'Where are you going to sleep, Daddy?'

'At Grandma and Grandpa's house,' he replied.

It seems odd, looking back, to see that I asked questions about my father's personal plans while accepting without question the plans for me. He would not be close anymore, so I expect I was scared, but it did not occur to me to say so.

I think by then I felt a bit dead inside.

The 'After' Time

The Stucco Bungalow

I suppose that car journey marked the beginning of another paragraph in an already fractured childhood. How long after my mother's death this was, I do not recall; perhaps a month or two.

Auntie Doris and Uncle John lived in a stuccoed bungalow. (I came to know those walls well because there was a very slippery path leading around the building to the back door and every time I fell I seemed to scrape my hands and elbows on the stucco.) I was taken to the spare room. There were only two bedrooms: both had double beds, with satin counterpanes, pretty curtains and a smell of paint. I do not remember feeling anything at all— just an acceptance, as I watched Daddy bring in my clothes and the few toys that had come with us. Then he went, exhorting me to be a good girl. He said he would come to see me and perhaps take me out the following weekend. The dead feeling might have increased a little as I saw him leave, but there was no time for thought or tears as Auntie Doris addressed me firmly.

I was told that there were rules in this house. Mummy had apparently allowed me to get away with too much, and now I would find things very different. At this point, the fog in my brain must have lifted because I know that I was scared. I sensed that neither my uncle nor my auntie wanted me there.

Daddy had gone away. Would he come back? Or would he forget about coming to see me? Did he want to see me? Daddy was always busy: would he be too busy to come next weekend, whenever that was?

I can now see that this whole scenario, of having to take on a small child, albeit her sister's daughter, was probably seen as a problem for my auntie. My uncle and aunt had only been married a few months; they were in their new home and were probably set for a year or two of quietly getting used to married life. I would have been an unwelcome addition to the household.

Auntie Doris already considered me over-indulged, and, who knows, perhaps there had been scenes and arguments between them. Perhaps my uncle did not want to take me on at all but had been shamed into doing so; maybe he did not consider the amount that my father was paying for my maintenance to be sufficient. From my adult perspective now, I can see that this was a difficult time for everyone and that I was the main problem. Taking me on, however, did not present one difficulty that such a commitment would involve these days: Auntie did not have to give up working or pay for child-minding (a concept unheard of at that time), as she had stopped working when she married, as most women did, to keep house for her husband.

A few days went by, and then I was roused early one morning and told that I was starting a new school.

But first Auntie Doris and I were to tramp across a field—it certainly wasn't school as I had known it during my brief attendance in Bath. We climbed some wooden steps to a timber building that seemed to have legs. Auntie opened the door, and I was amazed to see that it was, indeed, a school classroom. I was welcomed by a large man who turned out to be the one and only teacher of about twenty children of both sexes and all ages, from small to big. I had come from a tiny school of six girls run by two nice ladies in a large, smart house!

The class was made to say 'Hello' en masse, and I sat down at the front.

Then Auntie left.

Daddy came to see me the next day, which must have been a Saturday. I was in bed—in the big double bed—when Daddy came into the room.

'You not up yet?' he said.

'No, Auntie says—'

'She has a cold!' Auntie Doris took over. 'So she must stay in. You won't be able to take her out today.'

Daddy looked at me. 'You look all right.'

'Yes, I'm—'

Auntie Doris sounded firm: 'She is in my care and I think she should stay in bed.'

They left the room. I stayed in bed. Daddy came in later to say goodbye and then went, promising to return the following weekend.

I stayed in bed all weekend but was taken to school on Monday. Daddy came the next Saturday as planned, but this time I was deemed to have a sore throat. I seemed to be living on a diet of porridge. Once more Auntie Doris would not let Daddy take me out. I knew that he was cross, and he kept asking me about school, but Auntie said that I should not talk because of my throat.

However, when he came in to say goodbye, she was in the garden doing something, so she was not with him, and I remember we had a chat: I must have seemed all right, for he encouraged me to talk. I told him that the school had legs. After laughing at first, he looked puzzled and asked me more. It seemed that Auntie Doris had chosen the school: Daddy had not seen it and he did not seem happy with what I told him, probably about the building and the fact that we had a man for a teacher—most unusual for infant schools at that time.

I remember hearing raised voices in the living room just before he went and Auntie was very tight-lipped when she came into the bedroom.

I was taken to school on Monday as usual, but when we approached the field where the school hut was situated, it was full of water. It had rained heavily in the night, and some nearby stream or river must have overflowed. There were lots of parents and children there, looking at the marooned building. No one could get to it, so we went home.

Daddy came to see me on Tuesday. I was surprised—it was not Saturday. He wondered why I was not at school. Was I still not well?

'We can't get to it because of the water,' I said.

Auntie Doris must have been out; I know she was not there and Daddy was not pleased about the fact that I had been left alone. He stared at me, and I wondered if I had said something wrong.

'I want to see this school,' he said.

We waited for Auntie to return and then went to the school, which was still stranded in the water. Daddy was beside himself: he was so cross with Auntie for sending me to a 'wooden hut' instead of a 'proper school'. Those are the only words that I remember, but there were a lot of angry voices. Later, when Daddy came into the kitchen where I was playing, he said, 'You will be going to a decent school next week.' Then he left, banging the door behind him.

I think he must have arranged it then and there, for I have memories of being taken the very next day to a long, low red-brick building with a big playground.

Saturday arrived, and I was told that I had a chill and would have to stay in bed again.

'But, I'm all right, Auntie,' I protested. I must have gathered a little courage.

The Country Nurse Remembers

'I shall tell your daddy what a naughty girl you are, if you argue,' she replied.

I kept quiet but was still sent to bed, and I know I cried because Daddy would not be able to take me out. But this time when he came he was not alone. He had brought the doctor with him. He must have been unconvinced by all these so-called chills and colds.

The doctor looked in my mouth. I said, 'Ahh,' and then he listened to my chest, felt my tummy and asked me lots of questions. After a bit, he took Daddy to the end of the bed and I heard him say, 'I can find nothing wrong with the child. She is perfectly fit—rather thin, but . . . ' I don't remember any more and they left the room.

I sat in bed, wondering what was going to happen to me now. Then the door opened, Daddy came in and took my case down from the wardrobe, stuffed my clothes into it, gathered my dolls and books together, and then picked me up.

'We are going to Grandma and Grandpa's,' he said.

'I'm in my nightie, Daddy,' I objected.

Without answering, he wrapped me in a blanket from the bed and strode with me to the car. I was plonked in the front seat, and he went back for my belongings. No one said goodbye to anyone and we drove away.

Looking back over the years and trying to make allowances for the difficulties of being landed with a child to care for and the trauma of my mother's (her sister's) death, I still cannot see why my aunt should have wanted to prevent my father from spending time with me. One would have thought she would have welcomed a respite from the responsibility of a task she had not wanted and a break from a child whom I am sure she did not like.

Another puzzle was why she chose the wooden school with legs. It would have been a private school—perhaps it was cheap, less than my father was paying her for it. An unworthy thought, perhaps, but it is a mystery to me. By the time I was old enough to wonder and maybe ask about these things, the home situation was such that I was not able to ask my father anything about the time before my mother died or the time immediately after.

Perhaps I had not been a very good girl. I was five and had just lost my mother, who might have over-indulged me; I was with people who had no children of their own and who had their own ideas about my upbringing. They had their rules, but I was not told what they were until I broke them. In other words, I was lost and confused. I felt I had been moved from one place to another, from mother to grandparents, to aunt and to three different schools in a matter of months. There had been a lot of worrying shouting between Aunt Doris and Daddy. I had not had time to make friends, and I spent most of the time at home by myself. Did I get into mischief—real or assumed? Perhaps. Of course, I would have done or said things that would have been considered naughty and not known why. But I still did not think my situation strange. It just was. Had I been able to see the future, I might have realised that, in many ways, it was not going to change much.

So maybe my aunt felt she had good reason to shut me in the cold passageway by the back door until I learnt how to behave. I have no memory of what I had done on the first occasion, but I do know what I did to make Uncle John call me a 'blasted kid'.

He was trying to repair the wire to the back-door bell. This stretched round the outside of the house from the front door and must have had some sort of electrical supply. (Perhaps it was not the bell, but some other device.) I was standing nearby and was told not to touch anything while he went indoors. I thought he meant his tools, which he had left on the path beside me, so I decided to have a closer look at the wire that was running along the wall at just my height. I could see a break, and, being inquisitive, I picked up one end to look at it more closely. It seemed to bite me! I screamed and fell onto some cabbages by the path. I just sat there—probably dazed. My aunt and uncle came rushing out, hauled me up and marched me indoors. Back to the passageway! That is when I was called a 'blasted kid'. Perhaps I deserved it . . .

Having come so recently from Mummy's gentle and loving ways, I would not have really understood that I would have to live and behave very differently now. There were memories of my mother everywhere, which comforted rather than upset me.

Auntie Doris had some clothes that had belonged to her. A cardigan lay on the arm of the sofa one day—I had buried my face in it to smell Mummy's scent. It must have been her perfume—one that seemed to be specifically hers.

The sense of hurt I feel now is for the child I was then, trying uncomprehendingly to recapture a lost mother in the scent of her clothes.

After this discovery, I realised that there must be more things that had been hers, and so I sought them out whenever I was unobserved. I found some of her pretty dresses and a coat, and for a long time her scent lingered on them all. I can almost remember the perfume now, all these years later. It smelled like flowers. But, of course, the jumpers were washed, the coat cleaned and gradually even that tenuous link with my mother was lost.

On one occasion while I was still living at the stucco bungalow, I had just watched with sadness as another of my mother's jumpers, a familiar beige one, was taken from the washing basket to be ironed. At that moment I realised that her scent on that one at least would be gone forever.

'That was Mummy's, wasn't it?' I said to my aunt.

As soon as I had said it, I was afraid she would be cross, but amazingly she wasn't. She actually looked at me with a kind little smile and said, 'Yes, it was.'

Those were the kindest words that I remember her ever saying to me.

So maybe she was not the ogre I remember. Or if she was, maybe everything to do with her sister's death had been too much for her. I shall never know.

Even after I had grown up and was married, and I paid an occasional 'duty' visit, she seemed remote. Polite, but unfriendly. And I don't think she and Daddy ever spoke again after the day he took me away from the stucco bungalow . . . Back to a house that I knew well.

To Flossie's house.

To Grandma and Grandpa's house.

Return to Meadow View

Meadow View was at the end of a lane that ran beside the river for most of its way. Grandpa was the manager of the Works, and the house was the manager's residence. It had a big garden with a tiny orchard of about ten apple trees, a vegetable patch and lots of lawn. There were fields in front and behind it, and a weir roared past when the river was in spate or chattered quietly by when the water level was low. Sometimes there was so much water flowing that the weir became almost flat and the river overflowed its banks onto the field in front of the house. When this happened, the lane flooded as well and it was usually impossible to use it to get to the house or the Works, so everyone had to tramp up over the fields behind us, towards the village, which was on higher ground. This must have been a great nuisance to the grown-ups, but I thought it was fun!

The ground rose on the other side of the river, too, to form hills where the tiny village with the smithy nestled under a rounded, tree-topped outcrop. From Meadow View, we could just see the village church. There were a few houses on the opposite bank of the river, by the weir, and on our side there was only one bungalow, near the big gates that led to the

Works. Apart from these and our attached neighbour, the foreman's home, the place was isolated. I know it must have been quiet and beautiful, but to me it was just somewhere familiar, where Daddy had lived as a boy and where I knew I would be all right.

My father said that as we drew up in the car: 'You will be all right here.'

So I knew that I would be.

I have hazy memories of a house on a road higher up in our village. We had lived there when Mummy was still with us, but I must have been very young because I remember so little about it. There was a garden and a wooden garage where my father kept his Austin 7. I had a little friend next door and I recall playing with her, or perhaps just sitting and staring at her as she stared back at me, as very small children tend to do. That house would have been convenient for Daddy, as he was the assistant manager of the Works. Why we moved from there to Bath will always be a mystery to me.

Meadow View was just the same as it had always been on the day we arrived back from the stucco bungalow. I had been so afraid that something would have changed and it would not be so familiar. In fact, it was probably only a few months since I had been there, but that was before Mummy had died.

Flossie came to greet me, and I sat on the floor under the table, cuddling her. That table was used for dining, for playing billiards (it was so big) and as a den for me, Flossie and Crib—when Crib was not busy killing rats or chasing cats.

Grandpa was about to retire, so Daddy and some others had been building a house for them about halfway up the lane for when they moved from Meadow View. The new house, called Homelea, was built high up to avoid flooding, but this meant that there were lots of steps and terraces. There was much talk about how they should not have built it so high up; but I grew to love running up all the steps, round the terraces and down again. They were due to move in about a year, though I didn't know any of this as I sat under the table cuddling Flossie, believing that I was 'home'.

Aunt Lizzy

How could I not have mentioned Auntie Lizzy? She became a big part of my life for a while. She had been there all the time, with Grandma and Grandpa. Auntie Lizzy was my father's sister and lived with her parents at Meadow View. She had never married, and, when I was much older, I heard her sad story.

She was the only daughter and the oldest in the family. Even as a child she had helped Grandma, who was already going blind. They lived near Manchester when she and her brothers were young, and from the age of about sixteen she had worked as some sort of clerk with the local council. When Grandpa obtained the job of manager near Bath and the family moved south, she remained behind with an aunt because of her job. She got to know a colleague and eventually became engaged to him.

About that time Grandma's sight worsened so that she became totally blind. Meadow View, a fairly large house, had no electricity or gas, and with no modern appliances, such as a refrigerator or vacuum cleaner or washing machine, Grandma was finding it increasingly difficult to cope with two boys in their late teens and look after Grandpa and the home. So one day Grandpa wrote to Auntie Lizzy, asking her to come back. 'Your mother needs you!' he said. There was no thought for Auntie Lizzy's life and job in Manchester or her plans to marry.

The Country Nurse Remembers

My grandpa was the product of a Victorian upbringing and wielded a rod of iron on his family. My father and his brother had felt 'the belt' many times. Auntie—never! But the iron will behind the iron rod brought her back from her fiancé and her roots in Manchester.

By the time I was around, she had been living at Meadow View for many years, helping Grandma to look after Grandpa, the 'boys' (until they left home) and the house. She also worked in Bath for the council's rates department and travelled five or six miles by bus each way, with a thirty-minute walk to the bus stop, often coming home at lunch time to make her parents something to eat and rushing back for the afternoon. The fiancé had faded away when she had moved back. Perhaps his job prevented him from following, but she probably had to choose between marriage to him and her duty to her parents. Whatever the reason, she remained a spinster to the end of her days. She was loyal to her parents, loving her mother and obeying her father, always sure that her two brothers could do no wrong and protective of her nephews and nieces. She was fussy and nervous, but she always had the best interests of the immediate family at heart. This did not always suit her brothers' wives!

She would occasionally take a holiday with two other 'maiden ladies', as she called them, but apart from those rare times her life was one of duty and caring. I think Grandma probably appreciated her, but all the men accepted her role as the unmarried daughter whose job it was to look after the parents. She got little thanks. I didn't know all this when I was young, of course, and just accepted her as another aunt, but one who was very much a part of my early life.

Although single and childless, she coped with frequent visits from my uncle Jake, his wife and my four (later five) cousins, producing meals for all, getting beds ready, trying to join in the conversations but never having time—and looking after her parents as usual. Now she was suddenly, and without warning, presented with me.

Apparently, my father's decision to remove me from the stucco bungalow had been a spur-of-the-moment thing: understandable in the circumstances, but, with no telephone at the bungalow, he was unable to let Auntie Lizzy know that he was taking me to Meadow View.

I know she was not there when we arrived: she was probably at work. What a shock it must have been when she got home to learn that the care of a child had been added to her burden! I remember a great deal of worried discussion among the grown-ups about how she would manage and what would happen to me when she was at work. She would have to leave me with a disabled grandfather who was trying still to work himself, although only part-time—my father made up the time for him—and a blind grandmother. Would Grandma be able to cope with having a young girl, whom she could not see, running about the house and garden? Grandpa's disability made him frustrated and short-tempered—how would he deal with a small child on an everyday basis?

By this time, I was about six. I do not remember a birthday, but there must have been one somewhere among all the chaos. I do not know why I did not immediately start attending the local church school; it was perhaps the problem of getting me there. It was in the village beside the church and the manor house and was nearly a mile distant, most of the way alongside the river. With Grandma blind, Grandpa disabled, Auntie working, Daddy doing his own job and half of Grandpa's, building the bungalow and finishing Homelea, it was probably impossible for anyone to find the time to take me to school. They must all have known that the situation could not continue as it was.

Daddy and Mildred

While I was living at Meadow View with Grandma, Grandpa and Auntie Lizzy I became aware that something was going on that I didn't understand, and, because of snatches of conversation and a general feeling of unease, I started to feel worried. Something was going to happen . . . But did it involve me? I think I was beginning to realise that most things that caused the grown-ups to have whispered conversations usually concerned me.

I heard Auntie Lizzy say to Daddy, 'It's too soon. It's not right.'

Daddy usually had his meal in the evening with us all, but now sometimes he wasn't there.

Grandpa would say, 'Huh! Out again?'

I knew he didn't like Daddy going out. Grandma did a lot of tutting, and Aunt Lizzy looked worried. Then one day there was a lady there when I came in from the garden.

Daddy said, 'This is Auntie Mildred. Say "Hello".'

I was sure that I didn't have an Auntie Mildred, but there seemed to be so many aunts that I was probably unsurprised to meet another. I would have done as I was told (I almost always did) and was then sent into the garden again to play, while the grown-ups talked. After Daddy had taken Auntie Mildred back to her home, Grandma asked the others what she looked like.

'All right,' was all Grandpa had to offer.

Aunt Lizzy said nothing.

What seemed only a few days later Daddy took me to a house in Bath. Aunt Mildred was there, with two old people who turned out to be her parents. They were told who I was and asked me a lot of questions, which I tried to answer, but it was all about things that I knew nothing of: town things. Every time I stopped speaking, there was a long silence. Nobody seemed happy.

It seemed only a week or two later that we were suddenly sitting at a table in a hotel in Newquay. Daddy, Auntie Mildred and me. We were on holiday, I was told.

I recall we spent a lot of time on the beach, so it must have been nice weather. Then we would return to the hotel and wash and dress nicely to have tea—only they called it 'dinner'. Then we'd go for a walk along the front. Lots of people did the same, all nicely dressed. I shared a room (and a double bed; there were no twin-bedded rooms then) with Auntie Mildred, while Daddy had a little room right at the top of the building. He showed me the view from the window: sea, rocks and sand. Sharing a bed with Auntie Mildred was not fun like sharing with Auntie Jinny, who would laugh and cuddle and chat. Auntie Mildred came to bed very late and slipped in so quietly that I often didn't know that she was there until the morning. I wished it were Auntie Jinny instead.

Then the holiday was over and we all went back to Meadow View, before Daddy took Auntie Mildred home to Bath. We were telling Grandma, Grandpa and Auntie Lizzy all about the beach and the hotel.

'Mary slept with me,' explained Aunt Mildred. 'Maurice had a little room on the top floor.'

I joined in. In that moment I banged the first, and by far the largest, nail in the coffin of any hope that I might have had of a little affection from Auntie Mildred. And I didn't know how *very* important that was going to be!

'Yes,' I said. 'Daddy slept all by himself. Auntie Mildred and I slept together, but on the last night Daddy and Auntie Mildred slept together and I slept alone.'

There was a gasp and then a stunned silence.

Auntie Mildred turned, 'No, you didn't. We didn't. You . . . '

Daddy took a deep breath, 'Mary fidgets about in her sleep and Mildred was tired, so I slept with Mary to give Mildred a good night's sleep. Mildred went up to my room.'

'Yes, yes. The child is mistaken . . . ' Auntie Mildred was very red. She was stammering. Daddy looked straight at me and said, 'I was with you.'

I was frightened. I had said something awful. But what? I must have looked puzzled. Daddy said, 'You were asleep when I came to bed and still asleep when I got up, so you thought you had been alone.' Daddy always rose very early.

I was sent out of the room, and the grown-ups stood in silence for a while. The door was not shut, and I heard Auntie Lizzy say, 'Why would the child say it, if it were not true?'

Daddy turned and shouted, 'I have told you why she said it. She thought she was alone because I had got up and gone down before she woke. Mildred and I did not—repeat, did not—sleep in the same room.'

He took Aunt Mildred home without saying goodbye to me. She just frowned as she passed me in the garden. I sat and cuddled Flossie. I had done something awful but obviously had no idea what. Why was everybody so upset about it?

It must have been a terribly embarrassing moment for my father and Auntie Mildred. And at least at first no one seemed to believe them. In the long term, it did a great deal of damage to me rather than to them, as everyone believed them eventually. My father must have been furious at the implication, as he was a pillar of rectitude about such matters. The episode was not raised again in my hearing, and for a short while things seemed to be returning to normal at Meadow View.

A New Mother

One September day, Daddy said to me, 'We will be moving in to the bungalow now that I have finished it.'

I must have had an idea that something different was planned because I asked, 'Is Auntie Mildred coming to live there, too?'

'Yes,' said Daddy. 'Mildred and I were married this morning. We shall go to the bungalow today, and I will fetch you tomorrow.' He smiled. 'So you had better start packing up all those dolls, hadn't you?'

Out of kindness, various relatives had given me presents at the time of Mummy's death, and everyone seemed to have decided that a doll was the most likely thing to interest me. So now I had about ten dolls of various shapes and sizes, though Margaret was still my favourite.

Daddy gave me a great big hug and said, 'Now we are going to be a proper family again.'

I know I would have accepted this and the marriage and the move without question, but of the move itself I remember nothing, and the first few days of life at the bungalow are a mystery to me. I wonder, now, how my father felt about having built the bungalow for one wife and then taking a different wife to it. He was not an imaginative man—he was intensely practical—so I think he would have just done it.

Suddenly, I was going to school again. Daddy took me to the church school in the village on the first day of the autumn term. All my life, I have been glad that I went to that little school. It gave me a grounding in Christian principals and the Christian code of behaviour, as well as a good early education in basic subjects. This meant that I was able to get a scholarship to a Grammar school at the age of eleven.

I think Auntie Mildred took me to school for a few days, too, and then I was deemed to be able to go by myself. I was admonished to walk on the side of the lane away from the river and to go straight to school and come straight back home again. I must have had some catching up to do, as, except for my short experiences at the dame school, the school on legs and the red-brick school—none of which lasted more than two weeks—I was almost a year late in starting school. Although I did not have an enquiring mind, I did have a retentive memory, and this must have helped me to make up the shortfall in reading and writing, but I remember that when it came to sums it was always a struggle.

Looking back down the years at that tumultuous time, I can see why my father's hasty remarriage, less than a year after my mother's death, was never going to be idyllic. And it was all because of me: the problem.

In his early twenties, before his marriage to my own mother, my father had had a group of friends in Bath with whom he and Uncle Jake would go dancing or to the cinema; the pictures, it was called. My mother, whose name was Phyllis, and Mildred were part of the same group. They all had good times together, and eventually Daddy and Mummy married. At the time of my mother's death, Mildred was one of the very few women from that group not already married. And she was twenty-nine. In the days of the '30s and '40s, almost every woman wanted to marry, have a home and perhaps a family, and if she reached thirty without doing so, she was often considered to be 'on the shelf'.

The Country Nurse Remembers

Spinsterhood was something to be pitied in those days. Aunt Lizzy, for instance, was always 'Poor Lizzy'. So Mildred was probably delighted when my father started to take notice of her. Did she pause to think, here is a widower with a child and I am about the only woman that he knows who is not already married? Did she not wonder if he really only wanted a mother for his child and a housekeeper for himself and his home? Or did she persuade herself that he had suddenly fallen in love with her at that very convenient time?

And did my father not stop to think that there might have been alternative ways of looking after me (perhaps involving more input from him) rather than rushing into a marriage so quickly? Did he not think that this remarriage might alienate him, and therefore me, from Mummy's family and from most of the friends and neighbours who had known him then?

The answer is no. To my traditional and unimaginative father, who was also worried and bereft at the time, a new wife was the only way. Did he, perhaps, make it fairly plain to Mildred that part of his interest in her was to do with me? He was an honest man. But perhaps she realised all this without him saying so.

All this sounds very Freudian and cynical, but even taking me—the problem—out of the equation, it was not likely that the marriage would have been entirely made in heaven. Mildred was probably lonely. She had lived in town before they wed and had worked with a cheery bunch of girls and had fun with them. Now she was in the country, with a man who worked long, hard hours, living in a bungalow beside a river (she disliked the water), and instead of starting her own family with a baby, she had a ready-made family to adopt.

Added to all this was the fact that my father was demonstrative towards me and liked to sit me on his knee. Mildred gradually became very jealous, perhaps sensing that she came second in his affections. In subtle ways, she began to diminish this relationship, and I wonder now if jealousy was at the root of everything that happened from then on.

It was many years, however, before I realised any of this; in fact, I would have been almost an adult when I at last began to question, in my mind, why things were the way they were.

Life at Daddy's Bungalow

There was a lawn in front of the bungalow and a short driveway that led down to the narrow lane beside the river. The back door was at the side and led inside into a small passageway. This, in turn, led through into the living room, which had windows facing the river. The little kitchen, which we called our 'kitchenette' because it was so small, and the tiny bathroom opened off this room. The two bedrooms were at the back and were rather dark, the steep garden cutting out some of the light. There was another room, accessed from the front porch and called the 'sitting room'. Daddy levelled off a small patch in the steep back garden and grew some vegetables there, but it was quite a climb to get a cabbage or a few carrots. That was my job, and I loved it because I could see right over the top of the bungalow roof to the river and the hills.

From the windows or the front garden, I used to watch 'the chaps', as my father called the men who worked for Grandpa, go home on their bicycles. When I saw them, I knew that it would not be long before Daddy came home, too—perhaps on his bicycle or maybe in the blue Ford that we called Bluebird. I decided to wait for him outside the gate, on the grass verge, so that I could see along the lane.

'What are you doing out there? Come into the garden at once,' Aunt Mildred shouted from the window.

'I'm waiting for Daddy,' I replied, in answer to her question.

'I don't want you running about in the lane. Just come into the garden.'

Puzzled, I walked the five or six steps back into the garden and stood on the lawn. I couldn't understand. I had not been 'running about', I had been standing still. And I had just walked all the way home from school down that lane. But my instinct warned me not to mention this, and I just waited in the garden from then on.

Some months passed, and then it was Christmas 1937, our first in the bungalow. Aunt Mildred and Daddy put up the trimmings—I remembered doing this with Daddy and Mummy the year before, and I was sad when I thought back to the laughter we had shared. This year, it was all done after I had gone to bed.

In the morning they told me to go into the sitting room, and they stood in the doorway, watching me. I looked into the room but could not see anything unusual.

'Don't you like the tree?' Daddy said.

It was then that I spotted a small Christmas tree, which they had obviously trimmed with glass baubles, but there were no lights on it (we had no electricity at the time). It was on a fairly high table, and, from my height, I had not seen it at first. I was delighted when I saw it and must have shown it, but Aunt Mildred did not seem pleased.

'To think,' she said to Daddy, 'that we spent all that time on it and she didn't even notice it.'

Daddy looked at her and said, 'It is above her line of vision.'

He seemed rather surprised, too, and because I didn't know why, I imagined that it was my fault in some way.

During the first few months at the bungalow, I called Mildred 'Auntie', but now and then I forgot and said, 'Mummy' instead. Perhaps the threesome set-up reminded me of the time when it had been three of us before. I don't know—even now. So Mildred asked me if I wanted to call her 'Mummy' or 'Auntie' and said that I should make up my mind. I felt that she wanted 'Mummy', and by then I was beginning to realise that it was best to do what Auntie wanted. Also, I wanted to feel more like the children at school who talked of their 'mummy' saying this or 'mum' saying that. One or two had taunted me with a cruel sing-song: 'You haven't got a mummy, you haven't got a mummy.' I crept off at these times and cried in the lavatories. I didn't tell anyone—neither teachers nor Daddy nor Auntie—about this.

But still, surprisingly, I told Auntie that I would make up my mind soon. Equally surprising was the fact that Daddy had said it was up to me, although he must have known that Mildred wanted to be called Mummy. Could he have been thinking of my mother? Perhaps he was uneasy with yet another act that would separate her time from the present? Had he begun to think, after the initial excitement of a new marriage, that he had been indecently hasty? No one will ever know.

So, given the opportunity to make my own decision (I think it hardly ever happened again), and wanting to conform at school and feeling that I was expected to please at home, I decided to call her 'Mummy'. As soon as I said so, however, I regretted it. It didn't feel right. But I could do nothing because I didn't know how to describe the feelings inside me. I knew instinctively that it would displease Mildred, and perhaps Daddy too, if I told them that I had changed my mind.

Everyone accepted the decision. Those at Meadow View said very little, and I didn't know if they thought it a good idea. I'm sure Mummy's family would have been hurt and disapproving, but we hardly ever saw them now. But, for once, it felt like I had an opinion of my own and was not afraid to voice it.

After a few days, I suggested, 'Perhaps it would be more grown-up for me to say "Mum" like the bigger children do?' That felt better. And by that stage I knew that Mildred and Mummy were very different people.

I think it was at about this time that I began to imagine what it would be like to have a sister. I used to make up various scenarios where she and I would play together, even have adventures and sleep in the same room and giggle and tell each other secrets. I knew other girls who had sisters—perhaps older ones—and they seemed to have fun with them.

I was chatting away to this imaginary sister one day, thinking that I was alone, when Daddy came in.

'Talking to yourself? First sign of madness, they say!' he laughed.

'I'm just pretending that I have a sister to play with,' I said. I didn't want him to think I was mad!

Daddy stood quite still for a moment, then he said, 'You did have a sister.'

I looked at him, not understanding. I was an only child, I knew that.

'When your mother died, she had just given birth to a little girl. She died, too.'

I went hot all over. I had had a sister! She was dead! Just then, Mum called and Daddy turned away. My sister was never mentioned again.

Although I was sad to think that I would never be able to play with her, and I knew I could not ask questions about her, I hugged the news to myself. I had not always been an only child.

The Great Flood

So we come to the time of the big flood. The river that ran on the other side of the lane was prone to flooding, but this year it was on a Noah's Ark scale. The brown, swirling water rushed down the widened river and overflowed onto the lane. It came in at our gate and onto the lawn. Then gradually it crept towards the bungalow. We were not in any danger because the garden sloped up to the building, then the front door was at the top of a lot of steps, and there was another step to the inside—and so we stayed dry, but marooned. The steep back garden rose to some vertical rocks, with a hedge on their summit. Behind this were fields stretching away to the village, so Daddy came and went by climbing up the garden and out over the fields. From the windows, Mum and I watched the water in the garden and the swollen river. I thought it was all great fun, as I saw tree branches, hay bales, boxes, a shed and all manner of rubbish hurtle past in the foaming brown water. Mum was frightened, but I couldn't see why. We were warm and dry, Daddy brought in whatever we needed, and our coal shed was full.

In the field on the left of the bungalow, there was a wooden house. It was built quite close to the lane and therefore on lower ground than the bungalow. Because of the risk of flooding, it had been built on sturdy wooden stilts in much the same way as the school on legs, with a sort of short staircase up to the front door. There was another one a little farther along the lane, occupied by old mother Weston, an old lady who hobbled up and down the lane day after day. I once asked Daddy why she spent all her time in this way. He said that she had nothing better to do. I wondered what she ought to be doing instead but never found out. I remember her as being very talkative, and, looking back now, I can see that she was just looking for company as she plodded to and fro.

A very, very old man with a beard, Mr. Shepherd, lived in the first wooden house. He kept chickens on a tiny island a little way down the river towards the weir, which was opposite Meadow View. Every morning and every evening he would get into his wooden rowing boat, push off from the bank and partly row and partly paddle down the river to his island to feed the chickens and collect the eggs. The island was just out of our sight from the bungalow. I was sorry about this, as I would have liked to watch him feed the chickens. Now, with the water so high and flowing so fast, we were sure that he would not attempt this trip, but he did. He obviously knew the river well and steered a course towards the opposite bank, being battered by some of the floating rubbish but managing to bounce off and paddle downstream at a frightening pace. Sometimes the current spun him right round. Mum and I would watch him from the window, worrying that he might fall out or be swept away. He would disappear round the bend, and we would wait to see him return. It always seemed to take too long, and on one occasion he was out of sight for so long that Mum rang Daddy at the Works.

Daddy somehow managed to get from the Works to a place farther downriver, where he could see the island. There was no sign of old Mr. Shepherd or the boat, so Daddy waded along the lane to the nearby waterside pub to borrow a boat to try to find the old fellow. There, in the pub, wet but safe, sat the old man, taking refuge in the bar for a warm-up before braving the return journey. He refused any help, and we saw him appear round the river bend sometime later. By now, he was able to row across the lane, the water was so deep, and then tie his boat to the wooden legs under his house.

The next day, we saw him heaving two crates onto his old boat and setting off. It must have been earlier than usual because Daddy was still at home, having breakfast. Or perhaps it was a Sunday.

'The old chap must be going to fetch his chickens back here,' said Daddy. 'The island is probably flooding.'

He rushed outside to go with the old man to help, but he was too late. However, when the boat reappeared, sometime later, rocking wildly with the two crates strapped to it, all looking very precarious, Daddy waded out and helped him to unload and carry the crates, full of squawking chickens, to the higher ground at the back of his house.

I don't remember the end of the floods, or if all the chickens were saved, or what the garden or the lane must have been like afterwards, but I do remember the horses having to be rescued from their field near the river and being led to higher ground.

Daddy had come in, wetter than usual, saying, 'We've been getting the horses up to the top field. Their field and shelter is under four foot of water.' I was so glad that the horses were safe. How I loved those big Shires!

The bungalow was already connected to the gas mains, and at some point about then the gas pipes must have been extended to Meadow View.

The great big dining table that I used to play under was under the light. Aunt Lizzy had had to climb up to take down the oil lamp to clean the wicks when it started to smoke, then she had

had to climb back up again to hang the newly cleaned lamp; now, she just put new mantles into the gas light. I remember it being quite a business and much talked about: 'the wick needs cleaning' had become 'the mantle needs changing'.

I was with her one day when she was changing a mantle. I was asked to hold it and hand it to her when she was on the table. Unfortunately, I touched the papery substance, and, to my surprise and consternation, it virtually fell apart! These mantles were made of very fragile stuff, which looked like snowflakes, or the papery wasp's nest that Daddy had showed me one day. Aunt Lizzy was not cross; I just took another mantle from the box. Very carefully, this time!

At about the time of the flood, but probably not connected with it, something happened that meant that Grandpa had to retire. I understood that this meant he no longer worked and would therefore have to live in Homelea instead of Meadow View, which belonged to something called 'the corporation' and was for the manager of the Works. I expect Grandpa had had yet another stroke, or perhaps he had just reached retirement age.

So my father, who was already the assistant manager and actually did most of the manager's job to help Grandpa, became the manager, and we had to go and live in Meadow View. Mum was not very happy about this, as she liked the bungalow—not its waterside position, of course, but the small bungalow itself. I suppose Meadow View was a bit rambling in comparison and even farther down the lane. But I had been happy on our visits during my early years and foolishly thought that when we moved there this time, it would be much the same.

Oddly, again I do not recall the actual move. I know that, in addition to our own relocation, my father helped Aunt Lizzy to move all the paraphernalia of Grandma and Grandpa's years at Meadow View to Homelea. Mum helped, and I remember much talk about throwing things away and how Aunt Lizzy didn't want to get rid of things that meant something to them all. Mum was not sentimental, and she and Aunt Lizzy 'had words'. The first of many!

At last, we were there, and I had the little bedroom at the back that had been mine before. It faced the setting sun and was very hot in the summer evenings. I began to notice this, as I was sent to bed much earlier than I had been before Mum came.

But what had happened to Crib? He didn't go to Homelea with Grandma and Grandpa. And he wasn't still at Meadow View. He just wasn't anywhere. Flossie went to Homelea and sat in front of the fire there, but there was no Crib. The big kennel was still by the path, but Daddy soon chopped that up for firewood. Did I ask about him? I don't think I did. Possibly in my subconscious I knew that something horrible had happened. So I cried to myself because I had loved Crib.

All these years later, I am still sad to think that perhaps he came to an untimely end because his working days were over. If, indeed, this was the case, it proved to be a bad move, as there continued to be many, many rats at the Works—until they started to poison them.

Maybe Mum would not consider having Crib around when she moved to Meadow View; he was a very big dog, after all.

But how I had loved that dog.

Changing Times

We must have moved to Meadow View during the summer holidays of 1939, which means we had spent nearly a year in the bungalow. It did not seem so long, but my life was changing. People still did not tell me anything that was going on or about to happen, but where before I had been used to picking up snippets of news while the adults talked, now I was not allowed to play in the room when adults were discussing things. At Meadow View, there was a big sitting room, quite separate from the kitchen and dining room, and if the weather was not good I was sent in there to play, so I was excluded from hearing the grown-up talk.

If the weather was good, I was sent into the garden to play—usually with dolls but sometimes with books and pencils.

'Just take out what you want now,' I was told. 'I'm not having you running in and out all the time.' So I had to make up my mind what I wanted to play with and stick to it.

Playing or drawing alone in this way, I had not picked up at all on the worry that the adults must have been feeling, as world events were closing in—even in our remote corner of the world.

My memories of our first year in Meadow View are fragmented and probably entirely out of order. I was almost seven years old by now, and Mum had had a year to teach me how 'to behave'.

This was quite long enough to make me frightened of upsetting her, so almost all of my time at home was spent trying to please but not really knowing why certain things were deemed to be wrong. I was slowly adjusting to her discipline, her total control of my every move and, gradually, most of my thoughts, too. I know now that many of her demands were entirely unreasonable. But as a child I did not probe the 'why' but just did as I was told.

When Daddy used to have me on his knee, we both enjoyed a cuddle, but gradually this had to stop.

I remember one day Mum came into the room, glanced at us and said, 'Huh! At it again, I see.'

With a kind of common consent, I got off Daddy's knee and he put me down. As far as I remember, I was never to sit on his knee again. Why did he bow to these objections? I was only a child! Did he not realise that I was still bereft and needed love? Maybe he already realised that he had to do as Mum wanted to keep the peace.

One day, Daddy and Mum called me in to the dining room and sat me down facing them. They looked quite solemn, and I wondered, with that awful tummy ache that came when I thought I was in trouble, if I had done something naughty.

'We were thinking that it would be a good idea to call you by your second name, Julia, now,' Daddy said. 'Instead of Mary. You said there were lots of Marys in your class, so that would make things easier, wouldn't it?'

I was amazed. There had been no hint that any such move was being contemplated, and although I *had* said that there were five Marys in my class, I had never seen it as a problem. We knew who we were, I reasoned.

I must have remained silent because Mum suddenly instructed me to respond, insisting that she had taught me always to answer any question immediately.

'Um, yes,' I said, just to have something to say. This was taken as agreement, and that was that.

It took some getting used to. At home, I was Julia, and, at first at least, at school I was Mary, the subject of much sneering, as no one had ever heard of anyone changing her name. I was a 'show-off', they said!

Grandma was most disapproving and never called me Julia, insisting that I had been named Mary, so Mary I should remain. On the rare occasions that I saw Grandmother and Grandfather Radford, I did not even mention the fact that I was now Julia. I must have had some inkling that it would be unwelcome news to them. But one day Mum, who had taken me on a duty visit, was heard to call me Julia. They were very angry.

It seemed that the name Mary had been my mother's choice and her parents felt that her memory was being tossed aside. Mum was very tight-lipped as we went home that day, and she would not take me to see them again.

I have wondered over the years if the name change was, in fact, an attempt to expunge all memory of my mother. Perhaps not. To me, it was just one more change in an ever-changing life.

But these were small events in the general scheme of world affairs, and we were soon occupied by more important things.

The War Years

War

There was a big, wide, heavy back door at Meadow View. It was painted green and led from the kitchen into a porch, with shelves for shoes and boots, and on down three deep steps into a small yard. An outside lavatory, a coal shed and the lean-to greenhouse opened off this tiny yard.

One morning, I was coming out of the greenhouse with my quota of dolls or books for the day, which, I suppose, was to be spent in the garden, when Daddy came out of the back door, down the steps and into the little yard. His face was worried as he lit a cigarette.

He saw me and stopped.

'Don't leave the house or garden. We are at war with Germany!'

I looked at him, appalled. Not by the news, although it sounded frightening, but by his voice; it sounded so unlike the way he usually spoke. Then off he went to tell 'the chaps'. I was left wondering what this 'war' would mean. I was seven by now, but wars had not figured in my school curriculum. I did know that the term meant people fighting one another, but only from what had been read to me of the Bible.

I went back into the house to ask Mum what Daddy meant.

'Just go and play,' she answered. 'It doesn't affect you.'

I had to be content with this assurance, but I did not believe her. After all, Daddy had told me to stay in the house or garden. Why did I have to, if this 'war' did not affect me? (I was not allowed out of the garden, anyway.)

The autumn term began, and the grown-ups looked increasingly worried as they spent more time listening to the news on the wireless. Our radio was encased in a big polished wooden cabinet, about three feet tall, with patterns cut out of the wood at the front. It had to have accumulators (a kind of battery), which were huge and heavy, and we had to take them to the local garage from time to time to be charged up. Meadow View still had no electricity supply—it would be the 1950s before the lines were extended to the house and the Works—so everything was driven by gas or diesel generators all through and after the war.

I was told nothing about the war in lessons, either. The head teacher—we called her 'Governess'—would have received no instructions regarding the way to present the facts to under 11s, so it was hardly mentioned in class.

Not so in the playground, however. The boys, assuming a knowledge that they could not have had, started to tease the girls with tales of bombs and tanks and the imminent invasion by the wicked Germans. They were not alone in the belief that we were about to be invaded—most of the adults believed this, too.

Everyone was issued with gas masks in little cardboard boxes on strings and instructed to carry them at all times. We had a lot of fun in class, trying them on and laughing at one another. The boys chased the girls, trying to frighten them by making roaring noises from inside their gas masks. Everyone talked about air-raid shelters, and Daddy began to build a thick-walled concrete affair next to the back wall of the house. It had three bunk beds and a tiny table with an oil lamp on it.

The Country Nurse Remembers

We were told that the church bells would remain silent and would only be rung if there were an invasion. Thankfully, they were quiet until 1945, when they actually announced victory!

We heard for the first time the wail of air-raid sirens, as they were tested. And far away in London, plans were being implemented to evacuate children to the provinces, as fears of air attacks grew.

Evacuees

I don't remember the day our evacuees arrived, or the preparations that must have been made in advance, but suddenly two girls of about my age were there—in Meadow View. At first, I was delighted to think that I would have company. I was an only child and was not allowed to play with other children outside school hours. I made plans in my head for games that I might play with the evacuees. I also felt that Mum's attention might be split now, so that I was not under her perpetual scrutiny. Sadly, things did not work out like this at all.

The girls, called Lily and Hettie, came from a place called Poplar in the East End of London. I had trouble understanding them, and they must have found my Somerset burr equally peculiar. They were nearly two years older than I was and what we would now call 'streetwise'. I was in awe of their knowledge of London—or what I thought to be knowledge of London. Actually, they had rarely been outside their own area.

They knew nothing of the countryside at all and were always either frightened or scoffing of our quiet corner of Somerset. Hettie was terrified of the cows in the field next to the house—at first she did not even seem to know what they were.

'Cor, what's them?' I remember her asking Mum.

'Cows. That's where we get our milk from,' answered Mum, informatively.

'Coo. We gets ours from the milkman.'

Right from the start, I knew they would make Mum cross. They did not sit still at the table but got up whenever they felt like it and wandered about eating their sandwiches. Sometimes they would not come to the table at all: they'd just grab a piece of toast or bread and butter from the plate and run off. They did not come straight home from school but played with other evacuees in the village, and Daddy often had to go and look for them. They were amazed that anyone worried when they were hours late.

The first time Mum put a plate of stew and dumplings before Hettie, she said, 'Ugh! What's that muck?'

I held my breath, eyes wide, watching Mum. Had I said any-thing like that . . . well, I wouldn't have, anyway. I was scared for Hettie. But of course Mum could not smack an evacuee, as she would have done me. Oddly, I don't remember what happened afterwards, just the shock of hearing Hettie's words!

Lily was quieter than Hettie and seemed to have a little more idea about washing herself and eating at the table. One day, Mum asked Hettie what they usually had for their dinner at home.

'Dinner?' she said. 'I dunno. Mum just gives us a bit o' bread if we're 'ungry an' we goes out in the street. Or we 'as fish 'n' chips. We don't 'ave no table. Don't want one.'

I was told that I had to set a good example to them. I did not quite know what this would mean, so I just did everything the way I always had.

'Show-off! Snob!' was what greeted my uncomprehending efforts.

Hettie was soon in trouble in the village. She saw no reason why she should not leap over people's walls to steal plums or apples—or anything else that took her fancy—and thought nothing of pinching a comic from the village shop, Miss Mitchell's. The local policeman eventually got involved and appeared at the door one day. Luckily, Daddy knew him well and explained that these children were completely out of control and that he and 'the wife' were trying to curb them.

But Hettie and Lily just laughed it off. Because a telling-off was a dreaded thing for me, I thought that they would be upset, too, when it happened to them. But of course they didn't care at all.

One day in the orchard things went horribly wrong when I tried to play with the girls. I had always been allowed to pick the 'fallers' (fallen apples) and either take them indoors or, if they were rotten, throw them on the compost heap. I was not allowed to pick apples off the trees. Hettie and Lily started to throw fallers at each other and me, and when they had exhausted the supply of fallers they began to pick apples from the trees and throw those about. I hovered, whimpering, 'You mustn't!' but they took no notice. I started to gather the apples, good and bad, from the ground to sort them out.

Just then my father came stomping up the garden path, looking very angry. I had an armful of apples, and he must have thought that I was joining in the game. I was always scared of Mum's anger, but this time it was Daddy who was cross, and, without waiting to hear any protest, for the first and last time, he spanked me. It was through my coat and not very hard, so it did not hurt, but the injustice of it and the jeers of the girls did hurt. He could not spank them and they knew it, but he shouted a lot and made us all pick up the apples, put them in a basket and then go to bed.

Mum watched all this from the kitchen door and would not speak to us as we went in. Once in bed I cried bitterly, but Hettie and Lily, who shared a room, giggled and laughed and had some sort of play fight. I heard them with envy, but also with fear for them.

I never did tell Daddy that I had been gathering the apples, not throwing them about, but why didn't Mum tell him? She had been watching the whole thing from the kitchen door.

As the term continued towards Christmas, at first the village school ran in shifts. There were only two classrooms, and the evacuees doubled the number of pupils. Local children attended school in the mornings and evacuees in the afternoons. A teacher, Mr. Richmond, had come with the children and taught the evacuees. They loved him, and he had as pronounced an accent as they did. His classes were rowdy, and they all had great fun, as far as I could see. Governess was appalled at the 'lax attitude'—I remember those words, they impressed me.

Being a church school, we all went to church on Thursday mornings. Mr. Richmond had a row with the vicar because he did not see why 'his' children should have to go to church. I think he must have won the argument because I do not recall a single evacuee coming along.

I recall Hettie being taken to the school nurse when Mum discovered that she was wetting the bed. The nurse said it was the trauma of the evacuation and being away from her parents.

Daddy spoke to her that evening to say that we were sorry that she was upset at being parted from her father and mother. Hettie looked at him as though he were mad.

'Favver? That old bugger? I ain't sorry to leave 'im,' she said.

There was a shocked silence. I held my breath. What would happen now? My eyes swivelled from Daddy to Mum and back. I had never heard the word, but somehow I knew that she was swearing. Before Daddy could gather his wits, she went on to say that she missed her friends and the 'street' and that she didn't like the country because there was nothing to do and she was scared of the cows and sheep. She didn't like the food, and all the local kids were daft! The house was too big, and outside was too dark at night. And we had these funny lights—the gas lights. She liked going to the pictures, but there weren't any. And so it went on.

Eventually, Mum broached the subject of the bed-wetting again, saying that she would stop Hettie's bedtime drink, so that might help her to remain dry in the night. (I couldn't understand why the evacuees got a bedtime drink when I had never had one).

'What's the fuss? Mum don't mind if I wets the bed.'

'Well, I do. I have to wash the bedding every day.' Mum was very cross now.

'Wha' for? Mum don't.'

Another stunned silence. I tried not to think of a wet, smelly bed just left for days. I don't recall what the outcome of this conversation was, but the wetting went on.

Mum and Daddy showed great patience with Hettie and Lily, but one incident marked the end of their few months with us.

I had never heard of nits, but I was told that the girls had them because their homes were dirty. The school asked parents to treat all evacuees' heads, but DDT and other sprays had not been invented then, so as a precaution Daddy rubbed paraffin into our heads—*my* head included! Hettie shrieked and Lily yelled when Daddy rubbed the stuff into their hair, but they later boasted about it at school. I hated having to go there with my hair plastered down with paraffin in case the rest of the children thought I had nits, too—and was dirty!

I am horrified now to think of the danger. After all, we had open fires and a gas stove; our hair could have caught fire easily, but no one seemed concerned about that possibility; they were only worried about getting rid of the nits.

The paraffin was all washed off the next day, but it didn't deter the nits. They were soon in the bed, on their clothes and—the final straw—falling onto the table and into Mum's cup of tea!

That was it. First Hettie, then Lily was re-homed.

Hettie had several homes after ours, but no one could manage her, and in the end she was deemed uncontrollable. The final straw came when she set fire to someone's house. The authorities sent her home.

When I think back, I can see that Hettie was full of bravado. Did she even realise she was from a poor home? I don't think it even occurred to her.

Parts of her tale appalled me, but I was sneakily envious of the obvious freedom that she enjoyed. To be able to run outside whenever you wanted, to have lots of friends to play with, to be allowed to play in the street. We didn't have streets, we had lanes—but that would have been just as good.

Lily was much quieter and tried to understand what Mum wanted her to do, but it was naturally difficult for both of them to adjust. And in those days that was exactly what was expected of most of the evacuees. Very few allowances were made—they were to fit in to a lifestyle and surroundings that were utterly alien to them. Some of them were lucky and their surrogate parents were understanding, while many were better housed and better fed than ever before. Not all of them seemed to miss their home and family, and those who did soon went back, in spite of the danger of bombing raids.

There were just a few whose homes had been demolished and their parents killed and who, therefore, had to stay on until other arrangements could be made for them. Lily's parents, on a visit to their daughter, decided that they liked Somerset and eventually settled there after the war.

Gradually, many of the evacuees went home, as 'the phoney war' (as this period of calm became known) went on. People said it would all be over by Christmas, just as they had done in the First World War, and were disappointed when Christmas came and went and men were conscripted and the news was 'grim', as Daddy said. Not allowed to listen to the wireless or read newspapers, I could only rely on other children's highly coloured comments and opinions on the progress, or otherwise, of 'our side'.

Auntie Jinny Again

After Hettie and Lily had gone, Daddy decided that we should go away for a few days to cheer Mum up. She had certainly had a lot to put up with and much to do—with all the washing. It happened that Auntie Jinny had written a few weeks earlier, saying that she would like to see us, so off we went to the Cotswolds, where she lived. Petrol was already rationed, but Daddy was allowed some for his work-related trips and had managed to save just enough for this little holiday. How happy I was! I believe it was the first time that I had seen Auntie Jinny since my mother had died—two years ago now.

She hugged me with equal joy, greeted Daddy in her usual friendly way and made an obvious effort to be welcoming to Mum. But even I could see that it was an effort.

She would have disapproved of my father's hasty remarriage and seeing me probably brought her grief back, as well. But things ironed themselves out, and I felt loved and valued again.

Nothing seemed to have changed in the cottage, but there was something new at the front of the pub on the opposite side of the road. This pub was called the Corner Cupboard. Over the door was a flat porch with the stone head of a man on the top. At about this time a young man from the town had been called up and was about to go off to fight. His father had been in the First World War, and the lad still had his tin hat. On his last evening before leaving, he placed this tin hat on the stone head, saying that it was to stay there until he came home.

Tragically, he did not come home, but the locals left the hat there as a sort of memorial. Over the years, the top of the crown rusted away, and the 'brim' fell down round the neck of the figure. There it stayed for many more years until, eventually, it rusted away altogether.

Many years later, I learnt that the head was a bust of Benjamin Disraeli and that the pub had been a farmhouse, originally built in 1550. No one knows how it got its name, however.

Auntie and I went up into the town sometimes by ourselves. The buildings, round a sort of central square in the small town, were made of a lovely honey-coloured stone, and the pavement was several feet above the street, with some big trees overhanging the churchyard wall. I loved the high pavement; I had not seen one like it before. We went to little shops, and everyone seemed to know and like Auntie. We chatted about all manner of things, including Mummy.

'You won't ever forget your dear mother, will you?' she said.

'No. No, Auntie, I won't, but no one talks about her and I can't, either.'

'Why not, my dear?'

I could have said that I longed to talk about Mummy but did not dare. I didn't know what to say. When we were on our own, I asked Auntie Jinny lots of questions about Mummy. I was beginning to forget some things. Never her voice—that remained with me for years—but I could not remember what she looked like sometimes. Auntie had photos, though: lots of them! They were all black and white: colour photography had not arrived at that time. Some of Auntie's were so old that they were brown. I did not ask for any because they would just have been put away somewhere, but I just enjoyed looking at them and was happy when Auntie talked about Mummy to me.

Auntie and I were in the garden one afternoon, Daddy was painting a bedroom, and Mum had gone to the shops. I took a deep breath, then said, 'Auntie, I try to pretend that Mummy is still alive sometimes. But it doesn't work because there is this Mum, as well. Do you think Mummy minded going to Jesus? Wouldn't she have wanted to stay with me?'

Auntie looked upset but very kind, as she hugged me to her.

'Are you not happy, little one?'

'Oh, don't tell. Don't tell, will you?' I was in a panic. Why had I said that? Supposing Auntie said something . . .

But Auntie said, 'No. This is a little talk just between you and me. No one else. Now . . . I'm sure your mummy would not have wanted to leave you because she loved you so much.'

'Did she? I'm so glad!' No one had told me this.

'Of course she did, very much, and she didn't want to leave you. I know that. But she was very ill and God could not let her suffer, so she had to go. But I don't think you can pretend she is alive. It wouldn't be right. But you can try to remember all the things that you did together when she *was* alive. How would that be?'

'I'll try, but I was very small . . . Auntie, how do I know that she is happy with Jesus? I say my prayers every night and I ask God to bless everybody, but I can't ask Him to look after Mummy . . . They wouldn't like it. But she has the baby with her, doesn't she? My sister,' I added, with pride.

Auntie Jinny held me even tighter and gave a great big sigh. She probably had not known that Daddy had told me about my sister. She had tears in her eyes.

'I'll ask the angels to look after her when I say my prayers,' she said. 'It will be our secret.' She smiled, and I felt warm all over and not so worried about Mummy.

Whilst with Auntie Jinny, Daddy contacted Great Aunt Louisa, intending to take me to visit her. Great Aunt Louisa would have none of it. Daddy came out of the phone box looking very angry.

'She won't hear of it,' he said. 'She disapproves of Mildred and the fact that I married again.' This was not in Mum's hearing, of course.

Later, Auntie Jinny told him, 'Well, I'm not surprised. I don't want to lose touch with dear Phyll's child, so I try to ignore your behaviour, but . . . '

I held my breath. People did not speak to Daddy like this. What would happen? But nothing did because Daddy was fond of Auntie Jinny. Did he realise how much she and I meant to each other, I wonder? I cried when we left and so did she.

When we got home, I found that the arrangements at school had changed with the exodus of so many evacuees. Now we— the local children—were combined with the remaining evacuees. Why did Mr. Richmond stay when there were only about six of 'his' children left? Sometimes, he taught us all for reading. We found the class difficult, as he talked funny, we thought.

I remember one small London lad spelling 'drowned' as 'drownded'. Mr. Richmond said, 'It's not "drahhhnded", it's "drahhhned",' in his broad cockney accent. I'm sure he did not know why we all laughed.

Eventually, Mr. Richmond left.

Governess said, 'Now we can get back to normal!' This seemed to consist of our 'forgetting' nearly all that he had taught us and 'doing things properly again'. It was all very confusing.

Daddy would come home sometimes and say that so-and-so had been 'called up' and he and Mum would look serious. I knew that this meant that they were going to be soldiers, but I had no concept of what they would have to face: it all seemed so far away. Life went on as usual at home except that a number of 'the chaps' were called up, which left my father and the few remaining men very busy.

Will I *See* Again?

It must have been at about this time that I developed eczema behind my knees and ears. As young children, we all wore ankle socks, which meant that the lesions behind my knees became dry and painful in cold winds, but that mattered less to me than the fact that they *showed*. And with my hair being cut relentlessly short, the ones behind my ears were also visible. It was not until my mid-teens that these lesions cleared.

At school it was either 'Ugh' or 'Yuk' that greeted me. 'Is it catching?' some of the girls asked, while others just told me to keep away from them. It made me miserable. But there was little to be done to clear skin problems then, other than using a very sticky ointment that 'got on everything,' said Mum, and did no good anyway.

The eczema, and frequent streaming colds, bothered me for years. When I was sent to school with yet another heavy cold, Governess would be cross and send me home because I was giving it to all the other children. When I got home, Mum would be cross because I had to stay home the following day, and she said that I was just fussing. She did not seem to see my streaming eyes and red nose and my shivers. However, at such times or if I had a sore throat or had had a tooth out, and could not eat solid food,

The Country Nurse Remembers

I was given 'pobs'. This was a North Country name for broken-up bread mixed with hot milk and sugar. It slipped down easily, was sweet and quite filling.

Grandma—Dad's mother—and Aunt Lizzy had another recipe for people with colds.

Grandma used to say, 'Give the child a good boiling of onions.'

This 'good boiling of onions' was her cure for colds, flu, coughs, tummy ache, constipation and a lot of other troubles. It was not as awful as it might sound, as they were big onions, boiled with salt and a clove until very soft, then served with a dab of butter, or margarine in the war, or perhaps gravy. They made your eyes and nose run, but this brought out the cold, according to Grandma.

When I was about eight or nine, there was a severe outbreak of measles and mumps. Most children got these diseases by the age of about twelve, as there were no immunisations against them then and antibiotics, although already discovered, were not in general use until the early 1950s. Hopefully, you just got over whatever it was, but sadly these childhood diseases were often fatal or had serious and permanent complications.

One morning, I looked at my hands and immediately went downstairs in my dressing-gown.

'Mum, I've got spots.'

She looked at my hands and then into my face.

'Oh, my! You've got the measles.'

The doctor was sent for. I was a bad case. I was to stay in bed.

Over the next few days, I got worse. I could hardly walk, I was hot and cold alternately, I couldn't eat, could scarcely drink and the worst thing of all was that I could not see. I went quite blind. The doctor came and went, the curtains were kept closed and Mum had to lead me to the lavatory. I thought about Grandma and wondered if I was always going to be blind like her. This was frightening, but I was really too ill to worry about it. I think I was barely conscious a lot of the time.

The doctor seemed to be there a lot; various drops were put in my eyes, while some lotion was slapped on my spots. Mum was very kind. She washed me and helped me to drink some milky stuff, which was all that would go down my throat because the spots were even there. I was put in a darker bedroom because the light was bad for my eyes. Daddy came to see me every morning and evening.

Everyone must have been very worried about me, but, gradually, I began to get better and my sight returned, hazily at first but improving rapidly, and then I started to eat soft food.

I wondered if I had been almost ill enough to 'go to see Jesus' and, much more important to me, to see Mummy and perhaps my baby sister. Another thought came to me. Did Mummy know, away up there with Jesus, that I had been so ill?

The great day came when I was allowed downstairs to sit in the dining room by the fire in my dressing gown. Daddy had to carry me up to bed later because I was too weak to climb the stairs.

The illness lasted five weeks, and then I went back to school. Governess said I looked thinner than ever and should not have returned. A week went by, and I started to get a sore throat. The next day, I couldn't swallow, and my neck seemed to have disappeared altogether. My face looked as though it were part of my shoulders. I had the mumps!

The doctor arrived again. I was a bad case once more. I had been run down by the measles. My throat was so sore I could hardly speak. More staying in bed, more milky drinks, more hot and cold feelings and one big worry.

'Am I going to go blind again, Mum?'

'No. No. This is to do with your glands.'

The Country Nurse Remembers

What were glands? I had never heard of them. But it didn't matter: I was not going to be blind again!

Another three weeks went by, and I was deemed fit to come downstairs as before. This time, I tried to walk back up myself and was amazed to find that my legs would not work. Dad massaged them, 'to get some strength back into the muscles,' he said. I was given some nourishing white porridgy stuff from a tin, bought at the chemist shop, and gradually I got stronger and could walk properly again.

By this time, I had missed a whole term. I had not seen anyone my age while ill, and now I would not see any children because it was holiday time, with the isolation that brought with it.

But Mum had been nice to me the whole time, and I felt that made up for it.

Wartime Events

My memories of wartime events are probably fragmented and chronologically inaccurate; and, because of my isolation from any news of general events (I wasn't allowed to listen to the wireless), my awareness was on a personal, childish level. Inevitably, I overheard snippets of grown-up talk and opinions, but no one explained anything to me, so some of my ideas must have been based on nothing more than people's prejudice.

For instance, I overheard the grown-ups saying, 'The only good German is a dead one.' I was terrified by this language, so unusual in our home. In the playground rumours spread that the Germans ate the enemy's babies and that British pilots who baled out over Germany were shot on sight. Of course, if I had been older and had understood more, this would not have seemed so unlikely, given the pilot concerned had possibly just annihilated an entire German family. I expect the same happened in reverse, when Luftwaffe pilots landed in our countryside. But everyone was encouraged to believe that 'our side' was above reproach.

The boys at school sang some very rude ditties about Adolf Hitler. As a young girl, and having no brothers, I had little knowledge of the male anatomy, so I thought perhaps all German men were different in some way from our own men. Later in the war I was understandably baffled to meet some German prisoners who seemed quite normal! Of course the stories that I heard about Hitler's treatment of the Jews, whom I had previously only met in the Bible, proved to be all-too-true, but no one knew much about this until the war ended.

Dunkirk came and went, and the Battle of Britain took place. There was no possible way that I could have missed at least some of the excitement, as it was talked about by everyone. 'Our boys' were shooting enemy planes down daily over Kent. We lost planes too, but not nearly as many as the Germans. I heard all this from the boys at school, who listened to the news every day and discussed it with their fathers and grandfathers. The little playground behind the church school was full of roaring boys racing around, with arms outstretched, being aeroplanes. None of them wanted to be engine drivers anymore!

As children we had no idea about the fear and the horror the airmen must have felt every day. To us, and particularly the boys, the pilots were brave and clever, and the whole thing was wreathed in a sort of glamour. The idea that these terrific men might be afraid was impossible: we were encouraged to believe that fear was weakness. This was the way many grown-ups thought, too. Much, much later I realised that if these airmen *were* afraid, they had to be even braver to do their job and so still more deserving of our admiration.

No one went to the seaside anymore because gun emplacements were everywhere and rolls of barbed wire were appearing on beaches. Big round metal tanks, about twelve feet across and four feet high, called 'static water tanks', were placed at intervals in Bath and other towns. These contained water for the firemen to put fires out in the event of incendiary bombs being dropped. The water quickly became stagnant and filthy, but this did not stop the boys from boasting that they had been to Bath and 'swum' in them. The girls thought that was disgusting.

Big, important-looking buildings and some shops had sand-bags piled halfway up the windows. To absorb the blast, Daddy said. I wondered why they thought the blast would only affect the lower half of the window: the top half was still unprotected. I supposed they had to let some light in, and so it was better than nothing. When I was told that people flung themselves on the floor if bombs landed in the street, I understood. Most houses had sticky tape across the window panes in criss-cross patterns so that if the glass was broken by the blast at least some of it would hang together and it would not be quite so dangerous.

Notices were put up telling folk to 'kill that light'. The black-out had arrived! Mum made ugly black blinds for the windows and big curtains for the outside doors so that people could get in and out without showing a light—this was a pun-ishable offence, which sounded frightening, even though I had no idea what the punishment was. Even smoking a cigarette outside at night was now a punishable offence.

More posters told us that 'careless talk costs lives'. I was quite a bit older before I understood what it meant.

'Dig for victory' was the poster that most affected us. My father took this order very seriously, and every spare moment seemed to be spent digging up one of the lawns and planting vegetables. These spare moments were in the evenings: he was too busy in the daytime. I longed to help him, and, on the rare occasions that Mum allowed me to stay up a bit later, we dug and planted together. I always liked working with my father: gar-dening, decorating, looking after the various animals we kept. He did not talk much, but the silence was companionable. I was not afraid to talk to him. It was different from being with Mum. When she and I went shopping or to see her parents, I was always afraid that I would somehow say or do the wrong thing.

The Country Nurse Remembers

We began to see soldiers in uniform and others dressed as part of the Home Guard. For the first time, I saw people carrying guns. Even Daddy cleaned up the gun that he had used to shoot rabbits and said that he would be ready for 'any Jerry who tried to get into our house'. It all seems so haphazard to us now, but no one knew what to expect. They only had the First World War on which to base their knowledge, and there had not been the same threat of invasion then.

I began to hear the word 'conchie' used with contempt. I had no idea what it meant, but it seemed to apply to people who would not fight. I got the idea that these folk were tall, yellowy and ugly. Why? They were also strange and cowardly, and some people were attacking them. I knew nothing about 'conscience', and 'principles', and 'pacifism'. After the war was over, however, we began to hear of these so-called cowardly people rescuing wounded soldiers while under fire, driving ambulances in the bombing, digging trapped children out of collapsed houses. Then people around me went very quiet about 'conchies'. So they were brave after all; they just didn't want to kill people.

The period of the 'phoney war' seemed to be over, but 'our' war had not even begun. Where we lived was equidistant from Bath and Bristol. Both towns were to take a terrible hammering during the bombing, and while our village escaped lightly, we were on the noisy, frightening edge of these attacks.

But much would happen in my small life before those nights and days.

Hay and Fire

Meadow View was surrounded by fields. Sometimes there were cows in them, and I loved to see the little calves having a drink from their mothers. But more often they were kept for hay crops to feed the cattle in the winter. Haystacks were the preferred method of hay storage, and the farmer who owned the field bordering our garden built the stacks near the hedge. On nice days in the holidays, I would watch from the garden as the men tossed the hay onto something called an 'elevator'. A horse, attached to a horizontal pole, would walk round and round in a circle, providing the power to turn all sorts of cogs or wheels to make the elevator go up and over to drop the hay on the top of the growing stack. Another man would stand up there, spreading the hay flat so that a house-shaped stack was eventually created.

I was very unhappy about the horse. He just had to go round and round and round for hours. Then I'd feel very angry because some boy, working with the men, would sit on the bar for a ride. Daddy said that the horse would not notice the extra weight, but I still worried that it made it more difficult for the poor old thing.

The first summer after we moved to Meadow View I used to stand by the hedge and watch the hay-making, and once one of the men (there were two or three grown-ups and several children) came over to the hedge and asked if I would like to come over and join them.

'You looking lonely there all by yerself,' he said.

'Ooh yes,' I said. 'But . . . I'll have to ask.'

'Ah,' he said.

I ran indoors with my request.

'Of course not!' said Mum. 'I won't have you mixing with them.'

I went back to the man.

'I can't,' I said, sadly.

'Why not?'

'I'm not allowed.'

'Oh. I see. We'em not good enough, eh?'

The way he said it did not sound nice.

'I . . . ' I didn't know what to say.

Mum shouted from the kitchen window, 'Come away from the hedge. Just sit on the bench. They won't want you bothering them.'

The man looked towards the window. 'It's all right, ma'am, we'd like her . . . '

Mum had shut the window.

The man looked at me and pulled a face. I hoped Mum had not seen.

The bench was just like the ones you find in a park, and it was the only garden furniture that we had. Very few people had more than just a bench, usually placed on a lawn. There were no patios then; in fact, I don't think I had even heard the word. Things like barbecues, patio heaters, garden tables and chairs, gazebos and sunshades were unknown, as were coloured pots and tubs. Gardens were mostly practical, for growing things, rather than for leisure. Lawns had to be mowed with a push mower—even folk connected to the electrical supply were unlikely to have an electric mower. I think there might have been petrol-driven ones, but they were few and far between. One of 'the chaps' was meant to come once a week to mow the lawns, but sometimes the grass would get very long and Daddy would eventually do it himself. I would ask him to make 'paths' of mown grass round and round and in and out so that I could pretend they were roads and run around them. Of course they had to disappear, as all the grass was soon cut.

So, on this day, I sat on the bench, listening to the shouts and laughter and watching the bustle. I liked to see them all when they sat in the hay to drink lots of tea from tin mugs and eat great big, thick sandwiches. I drew a sigh of relief when they unhitched the poor horse and gave him a drink of water from a battered bucket. To the children among them, it must have been like a picnic.

When the stack was finished (perhaps two stacks, if it had been a good year), it was left for a while to settle, and then a sort of straw thatch would be fashioned to keep it dry. When the winter came and the men started to use the hay, they would cut it out in big blocks from under the thatch until at last the thatch fell down and then that was used for animal bedding. Nothing was wasted in those days.

One year, after the haystack had been built, I was sitting in the garden when I began to smell burning. It had been a wet summer, and the farmer had not been able to get the hay really dry. The stack had been built too soon, said Daddy. We had seen steam rising from the stack when the sun was hot, but that particular afternoon I could tell the smell was different. I called Mum, who rang Daddy at the Works. He came home and rang the farmer. He arrived very soon afterwards, but the smoke was so thick by then that he decided the stack could not be saved. He was prepared to just leave it to burn itself out, he said.

The Country Nurse Remembers

Just then the wind changed and started to blow the smoke, and soon the flames, over towards our house. Mum screamed, and Daddy ran for the phone to ring the fire brigade. I was a bit scared, but very excited.

Soon the rattling red fire engine came clanging down the lane and pulled up beside the hedge. The men began to unroll the big hoses. They had to stand well away to hold them, as the flames and the heat were now very dangerous, so the water shot upwards in a big arc before landing on the hayrick, where it fizzed and spluttered.

'Mildred, get a few clothes and anything important together. We might lose everything.' Daddy was helping the men and shouted this over his shoulder.

'Fetch your clothes, Julia.' Mum was running up the stairs.

We gathered clothes and some photos and some papers, and Mum stuffed them in suitcases, putting them just inside the kitchen, ready to 'grab and run if I say', as Daddy had shouted. I made sure that Margaret was among my things!

At that time, people had far fewer clothes and other possessions than we do now, so a couple of cases were all that was needed for essentials.

Outside, the hoses were pouring gallons of water onto both ricks. Evidently, the second was smouldering and the smoke was now mixed with steam. The noise was frightening. The roaring of the flames, the swooshing of the hoses, the hiss of the steam and the crackling of the thatch were combined with the shouts of the firemen. Then the hoses were turned onto our shed, which was near the hedge. Daddy kept all sorts of tools and useful bits and pieces in there.

I suddenly remembered two toys that I had not seen for years. 'Where is Ted? And where is Wilfred?' I asked.

'What?' said Mum.

'Ted and Wilfred. I haven't seen them for a long, long time.'

'I don't know what you are talking about. In any case, now is not the time to worry about such things.'

But I *was* worrying. I had completely forgotten about these two once-precious toys and was afraid that they might be in the shed. But there was nothing I could do about it.

Very gradually the flames died down, the men scattered the remaining hay and straw, and continued to soak it all. The shed had survived, and our house was no longer in any danger.

Later that day, after the fire engine had gone and Daddy, black from head to foot from the smoke, had washed the dirt off, we were looking at all the mess, and I thought of Ted and Wilfred again.

'Daddy, what happened to Ted and Wilfred?'

Daddy looked at me, thought for a bit and then opened the shed door and rummaged around a bit. There, on a high shelf, looking rather wet and bedraggled, were the big teddy bear and the equally huge rabbit. How could I have forgotten these two? They had been so much a part of my early life. One or the other had accompanied me everywhere. Ted was a huge, fluffy bear with a very happy face, while Wilfred was a pink rabbit in the sitting position with very large, wired ears. He must have been about three feet tall. I remember that I could not carry him when I was small.

I was so thrilled to have found them again, but I have never understood why they had faded entirely from my mind until the haystack fire. And why I suddenly thought of them then.

The Plane Crash

We were becoming used to the sight of aircraft returning home from bombing raids on Germany as they flew over us on their way to the air base in Bristol. Often the plane was in a poor state, with holes in the wings where they had been hit by anti-aircraft fire. We could clearly see the sky through these holes, they were so big! Sometimes we could tell that one of the engines was not firing properly because the sound was all wrong, then the plane would fly lopsided, and often there would be smoke coming from the rear or from an engine. Occasionally, a plane was so low that we could see the pilot as he struggled to keep his crate, as the planes were called, in the air. Then we would hope that it got to the airfield safely. Sadly, some did not; we heard that several of the planes that we saw crashed before getting home.

We children were now able to tell by the engine sound if it was 'one of ours' or 'one of theirs'. Some of 'theirs' straggled home to Germany or France over our house, often in a very bad way. We ought to have been afraid because they frequently offloaded their bombs to lighten the aircraft so that they had a better chance of getting back—but we were fascinated, and bloodthirsty enough to hope that they would crash so that we could cheer.

But one afternoon it was one of 'ours' that crashed in the village.

Mum and I had been to the grocer in the middle of the village and had set off to go to the co-op. A plane, pouring smoke, came from behind us and roared over the village very low, almost touching two tall houses as it rapidly lost height, completely out of control.

Mum grabbed my hand to rush for shelter somewhere, but we did not know where to go; the plane was swinging from side to side and could have landed just about anywhere. We started to run, but I didn't know where we were going. Other people were rushing to and fro, as well. Then the plane lost so much height that it disappeared behind a row of houses, and a moment later we heard a terrific bang and a lot of crashing noises. By this time, we were crouching behind a low wall, but it was obvious that the actual crash had occurred at the bottom of the hill on the edge of the village, a little way off.

I know we had been going to do more shopping, but Mum was shaking and decided that we would go home instead. On the way down the lane, we met Daddy, driving up to find us and see if we were all right.

'I'll take you home and then I'll be back to see if I can do anything to help,' he said.

He was home again quite soon, as the ambulance and the fire engine were already at the crash scene, which was in the railway station yard. The plane had nose-dived into the weigh bridge, and no one was hurt except the pilot, who was 'very dead, poor chap', as Daddy said.

Later we heard that the plane had been involved in a dog-fight over Bristol. 'Dog-fight' was the name given when an enemy plane and one of our planes were involved in a battle in the air, shooting at each other and swirling and swooping to avoid the bullets. I thought dog-fight was a great name. I remembered Crib's dog-fights!

The Country Nurse Remembers

The enemy plane had crashed in the suburbs of Bristol, but our pilot had tried to avoid killing people on the ground by steering away from the town and our village.

'He could have bailed out, but he stayed at the controls to avoid bloodshed. The man was a hero,' said Daddy, who was most upset. 'He saved dozens of lives by staying put and steering that plane away from built-up areas. They say he was already wounded, too. I hope they award him a medal.'

I couldn't understand this at all. I didn't know that anyone could get a medal after they were dead. Where did they put the medal?

In the playground, everyone talked about the crash for at least a week. The boys pretended to be very knowledgeable about the type of plane, who the pilot was and what the dog-fight would have been like. Most of them had managed to get close enough to the cordoned-off area at the station to see the bent and twisted aircraft. Many claimed to have seen blood! We were all most impressed.

One of the boys, I'll call him David, had certainly been very close. A week or two after the crash, his mother began to notice an unpleasant smell about the house and could not identify its source. Then, one day, as she was turning out his pockets, which were usually full of bits of string, sticky crumbs, cigarette cards and the like, her fingers touched something smooth and soft. A she pulled it out, she realised it was the pilot's thumb! Her screams could be heard in the next road, apparently.

David, with the thumb in a tin box, was taken to the police station and given a good ticking off. But for days, of course, at school he was the centre of morbid interest. What ghouls we were! We wanted to know if 'it' was covered in blood. Was the bone sticking out? Was it a big thumb? Was it all there? The only thing that slightly spoilt the excitement was the fact that the pilot was 'one of ours'. 'Wish he'd been a Jerry,' was the general opinion.

Tig and Trouble

Two things seemed to happen at home at about the same time. We got a puppy—which was lovely—and there was a big family row—which wasn't.

Every Friday on the way home after school, I went to see Grandma and Grandpa at Homelea for about an hour. I hardly ever saw Aunt Lizzy on these visits, as she only got home from work just before I had to leave, strictly at 5:30 p.m. This particular day Mum told me to stay until she and Daddy came to pick me up at about 6 p.m., so Aunt Lizzy was at home and had given me milk and cake to keep me going until teatime, she said.

While I was with them, Grandpa started to ask me all sorts of questions. Aunt Lizzy kept trying to stop him, but he took no notice.

'What do you do when you get home from school?' he asked.

'I clean my shoes.'

'Then what happens?'

'I have my tea.'

'By yourself?'

'Yes, Daddy is not home by then.'

'What do you have for tea?' he continued.

'Bread and butter and jam or something, perhaps cake and a cup of tea.'

'Do you go home from school for dinner?' Dinner meant 'lunch'.

'Yes, except on Fridays.'

'Fridays?' he questioned.

'I take sandwiches to school for dinner and have whatever they have had for dinner, for tea. Mum puts it in the oven,' I explained.

They knew that Daddy had to go into Bath on Fridays to do something to do with the Works. Perhaps they didn't know that Mum went with him. So I stayed at school to eat my sandwiches. I was usually the only one.

'Then I do some washing up and then I have about half an hour to play in the garden, if it's nice, or the 'other' room, if it's raining, and then I go to bed.'

'What time is that?'

'Quarter to six, except Friday, like today.'

'What about supper?'

'I don't have supper. I've had tea.'

'I mean later, like just before bed.'

'No, I'm not allowed,' I said.

'What time was tea?'

'After school—half past four. When I get home. Except on Fridays.'

'What do you take to bed? Dolls, books, pencils?'

'I have to go to sleep,' I answered.

'And do you?'

I was scared here because if I said 'Yes,' it was a lie, and if I said 'No, I can't because it's too light and I'm not tired,' and they told Mum, I would be in trouble. I think I was about nine at the time and no one else I knew was sent to bed so early, so I was called a baby at school. I didn't know that early bedtimes would go on until I was at least thirteen and were only relaxed then because of homework. Oddly, I do not remember what my answer was in the end.

All through these questions, Grandpa kept giving Aunt Lizzy a 'look'.

'It looks as though she was right,' he said eventually.

Aunt Lizzy looked worried. 'Yes. She's been school nurse for a long time.'

In fact, a few days earlier, Nurse Furney had been to the school to inspect the children. Parents were not involved in this when I was at school: the nurse just turned up, and the children were marched in, one by one, to see her. They undressed to knickers or pants and were given the once over. The nurse was a friend of Aunt Lizzy. I began to feel worried in case I had said something to the nurse that would get me into trouble. 'Inspection day' was taken as just a bit of fun at school. Why were there all these questions now?

Then we heard the horn. Daddy and Mum had arrived. I ran down the steps to the car. There sat Mum with something under her fur coat.

'Look,' she said. She was smiling.

I looked. It was a brown-and-white puppy, very wriggly and squeaky.

I was delighted. A puppy! Now I would have someone to play with in the garden. I would be able to give him his dinner, walk him . . . I was so excited.

But then I remembered Peter-the-Pup.

He had disappeared.

And Crib. He had disappeared.

Would this dog vanish, too? Oh, I hoped not. I didn't want to love another dog, just for him to be spirited away.

We took him home. He had to be bathed, because he had been born in a dirty stable and his coat was full of fleas. Daddy brought the old tin bath in, and he was popped in and washed with carbolic soap. He didn't like this, and squirmed and whined. I was allowed to dry him on an old towel, and he licked my ears and bit my nose and wagged, not just his tail, but his whole back end, while I cuddled him. I was so happy!

Mum's coat was also full of fleas, and she screamed as she took it off. Daddy took it into the garden and shook it and shook it.

'What shall we call him?' I wanted to know.

Just then, he did a 'tiddley winks' on the floor.

'Let's call him Tiddley Winks,' laughed Daddy.

'That's too long,' said Mum. 'What about Tig?'

So Tig he was, and he lived with us until, at the age of about ten, he had to be put to sleep. I used to cuddle him and whisper to him, and he seemed to love me, too. He was much more than just a dog to the lonely, rather frightened child I had become.

The next day my father went to see Grandma and Grandpa. It was a Saturday, so Aunt Lizzy was there, too. He came home, called Mum and they both went into the dining room and shut the door. After a while and a lot of loud talking, Daddy called me. I knocked on the door and was told to come in.

'Why do you knock the door?' asked Daddy in a surprised voice.

'Mum says I must knock before I go into a room.'

He looked at her. 'Why? This is not our bedroom or any-thing.'

'I'm not having her barging in on private conversations,' said Mum sternly.

My father looked a bit taken aback, as well he might, as I never barged anywhere. In fact, I was a bit of a mouse.

'Oh,' he said, then told me to sit down.

What had I done?

'What have you been saying to Grandpa and Aunt Lizzy?' he asked.

'I . . . What . . . what do you mean?'

Mum spoke. 'It's a simple question. Just answer it.'

'Grandpa asked me lots of questions about my tea and bedtime and things.'

'You must have told him some lies then, because he thinks I am not looking after you properly,' said Mum.

I was sobbing by now. 'I didn't, Mum. I told him what I have and when I go to bed.'

'You must have said something to make him ask about all those things?'

Daddy interrupted: 'Just leave that, Mildred. What about the nurse's inspection?'

I didn't know what he meant, so I just looked at him.

'Why didn't you tell me that she had been?' asked Mum.

'I . . . I forgot.' It was such an ordinary event that I had forgotten about it.

'So. What did she say, when she looked at you?'

'She said, "Oh dear! What a pale, thin, quiet little girl you are."' I trotted out the exact words.

'Why did she say that?' Mum was very red.

'I don't know.' I knew that there was going to be big trouble of some sort.

I was not aware of the fact that I *was* pale and thin and too little. I was probably quiet as well, because home was still a place where, for the most part, I only spoke when spoken to.

Daddy was looking at me with a worried frown. Mum seemed to gather herself together. 'You'll have to eat more and get plenty of rest,' she said.

I must have suddenly gained some courage. 'But, Mum,' I said. 'I eat everything you give me, and I go to bed when I'm supposed to.'

Whoops!

Mum looked at Daddy and said, 'You see how cheeky she is!'

He seemed startled. 'But does she eat everything you give her?'

'Well, yes,' said Mum. 'I'll have to give you more, I suppose. But I don't want you overloading your stomach.'

'Overloading my stomach' was a favourite phrase of hers. If I was sick and certain foods affected me badly, or if I was particularly worried about something and had a 'bilious attack', Mum would say that I had 'overloaded my stomach'. After these events, she always cut my food down, not just for a day or two, but for about a week. But until that moment I had not realised that I was almost perpetually hungry. The revelation was a surprise. The constant feeling in my tummy was just that: the feeling in my tummy! I had not associated that feeling with chronic hunger.

Maybe I was going to get more food now, I thought—though Mum forgot that I had not had any tea that evening and I did not dare remind her. So again I went to bed with a rumbling tummy.

Food rationing had begun by this stage, but at first only a few things were limited, and because we lived in the country with vegetables and chickens, there was no need for hunger. But I was not allowed in the larder or to ask for extra helpings or to have more than my allotted meals or drinks. Snacking was certainly not considered.

Along with most children at that time, I was given a dessert spoon of cod liver oil and malt daily. It was toffee-like and gooey, and tasted of fish, but I loved it! Most school friends said 'ugh' and hated it, but it was quite filling, as well as being good for you. In the summer, it was considered to heat the blood too much, so Parrish's food was substituted. This was a bright red medicine-like liquid that tasted horrible. I think it was full of iron, which is also good for you . . . So I was probably all right for minerals and vitamins, just rather empty.

I don't think my father had given my appearance a thought. As with most men of that era, he worked and provided, while the upbringing of a child, particularly a girl, was the woman's job. Days would go by and I wouldn't see him, because he would be gone in the morning and still working after I had gone to bed. I do not think he noticed. As far as he was concerned, I was being looked after, and that was that.

There was a very stiff atmosphere with Grandpa and Grandma for a while, and I was not allowed to go alone to see them. Mum did not speak to me, except for essentials, for days. Being sent to Coventry was one of Mum's main punishments, and, with no-one else to talk to, I was very miserable.

But at least there was Tig now, and I could talk to him.

I knew that my mum was much stricter than all the other mums, but that was just the way it was. But now I began to see that nearly everything about my upbringing was different. I was often teased at school because I was not allowed to stand and talk to the others after school, as I had to leave immediately and walk straight home—alone. If I waited for my friends who lived farther up the lane, I might be late. I could not hover outside Miss Mitchell's shop with the rest, or pause to pick flowers. I must wear my coat, not carry it. I had to wear my gas mask (in its box) and my satchel in a certain way. As time went by, I began to realise just how many things there were that I must or must not do that seemed peculiar to the other children.

Being different from them made me miserable, and when they all laughed at me I was very ashamed. Unfortunately, I covered this with a sort of bravado, a pretence that I did not mind Mum being so strict or that it was my idea to do things in such and such a way. This meant that I was often described as 'weird' or 'daft'.

Why did I not admit that I was not happy with Mum's rules? Was it family loyalty? Or a kind of pride? I would not have known what all these words meant anyway, but my prickly attitude ensured that I was not all that happy at school. No one knew, of course, because no one asked me.

I was glad that they did not know what went on at home.

After hurrying home from school, I had to say 'Hello', then take my shoes off, put my slippers and apron on and clean my shoes. Then I went to the lavatory, washed my hands and wrists in the kitchen sink and wiped the bowl round afterwards, Mum watching and timing me. Then I sat at the table and ate my bread and butter and jam before I was allowed to drink the one cup of tea. I was often very thirsty in hot weather by the time I had hurried home, but I had to stick to this ritual. I always ate under Mum's eye but not with her or Daddy. I would then wash my plate and cup and saucer, wipe the sink round and go into the garden or the other room until quarter to six. I had to keep an eye on the clock and tell Mum when it was bedtime. If I forgot and was a minute or two late, there was trouble. It was difficult when I was in the garden, because I had no watch.

I would go upstairs and undress; everything taken off in a certain order. All had to be folded precisely and placed neatly on my chair. Then I put my nightdress on and went into the bathroom and brushed my hair, being careful not to look in the mirror. All this would not have been so unreasonable, but Mum timed me, and I was rarely quick enough to please her.

She would then hear me say my prayers, which followed the same pattern every night. Then the curtains would be pulled, and I would get into bed. Mum would say 'goodnight', give me peck on the cheek (or not, if I had been too slow) and go, telling me not to fidget about and to 'get to sleep'. In the summer, the sun shone into the room, and it was hot. I would have liked to move to a cool patch of the bed, but the springs squeaked and Mum would hear and shout up the stairs, 'Just lie still and get to sleep!' No dolls, no teddy, no books . . . just sleep.

It was worse when I had a cough because I was not *allowed* to cough! Mum said it was not necessary and I was just fussing, so I tried to stifle it. But it was usually a tickly end-of-cold cough and I couldn't stop it, so I got into trouble. If I had been allowed a drink of water, it might have been better.

In the holidays, I was not to get up until Mum called me, and that was often not until about ten or eleven o'clock, by which time I was starving, having had tea at four-thirty the day before.

One day I did get up and come down. Mum was so cross.

'I thought I would get up and . . . ,' I said.

'Well, you can just get off back to bed until I call you. And you don't need to think. I'll tell you what to think,' she shouted, and I crept away.

Sometime later (I think), Mum said, 'It might be as well if you don't tell people how late you get up. They might think you are lazy.'

I didn't want people to think I was lazy, so, as usual, I complied. Now I can see that she was afraid that people would hear that she made me stay in bed to be out of the way.

Once a year, in the summer holidays, I was allowed to have a little friend, Sheila, to play for the day. And once a year I could go to her house to play. I loved going to her house, as her mum gave us nice drinks and we could play indoors or out and have as many toys with us as we wanted. I was less happy when she came to our house because, apart from the restrictions, which I knew she would find odd, I was afraid that she would say something that would get me into trouble. Perhaps I had not worn my hat out to play in the playground (no one else did), or maybe I had stood on the wall to watch the aircraft. She might talk about this and then Mum would know, and, after she had gone, I'd be in trouble.

'Trouble' was not often just spanking; more likely it was being sent to Coventry, or Mum would tell Daddy that I was a naughty girl, or there would be some pushing or pulling through a doorway or up the stairs.

One day, she pushed me down the back steps for some reason—I think I had been slow doing something. I had in my hands a small, sturdy wooden stool. I fell onto it, and one of the legs went into my ribs. It hurt a lot every time I took a breath, but I went into the garden and sat on the bench. Mum must have had some idea that she had hurt me.

Later, she said, 'Did you hurt yourself when you fell?'

I could tell from the way she said it that it was going to be my fault, so I muttered, 'No.'

It hurt for several weeks, and many years later, an X-ray for something else showed a healed greenstick fracture of two ribs.

But sometimes Mum could be nice, even friendly, telling me tales of her youth and the fun that she and friends used to have. And when Daddy had time we would all go for a walk round the village with Tig, or perhaps Mum and I would watch him playing bowls—he was a county 'reserve' player, which I understood meant he was very good at bowls. Occasionally before petrol rationing and again after the war, Daddy would take us out to Exmoor or the Exe Valley, or to the sea at Clevedon or Weston for the day. So it wasn't all doom and gloom. But I always had to be very careful about what I did and how quickly I did it and what I said.

Tragedy

At the time we moved to Meadow View, Daddy let his bungalow by the river to a family called Anderson.

Mrs. Anderson wore long, flowing dresses and coats and looked very quaint. Mum said she was very odd. There were two boys about my age and a little girl, perhaps about three years old.

The boys were quite tough and roamed about brandishing sticks. One day they barred me from walking down the lane after school so that I was very late home. Mum thought I was making it all up, but eventually Daddy, who had heard 'no good of these boys', went to see Mr. Anderson about it. Mum just said that I should have stuck up for myself. I wondered how, when there were two of them, plus a couple of their friends, all with sticks, standing in a line across the lane.

But soon this family experienced a most dreadful tragedy. The little girl, Elaine, had a tricycle, and one day when Mrs. Anderson was inside the bungalow, Elaine rode her tricycle too near the river's edge and toppled in. No one saw: no one knew. And she drowned.

The whole village was shocked and blamed her mother for allowing her near the river on a tricycle at the age of three. My parents were outwardly sympathetic, and Daddy did what he could, but he said that Mrs. Anderson was 'not right'. Grandma and Grandpa, next door in Homelea, could not understand 'that woman', and there was much discussion about the generally odd lifestyle of the Andersons.

Some months later we were told that Mrs. Anderson was going into hospital. No one mentioned breakdown, or mental strain, or depression—things like that were not spoken of in the 1930s—but she must have recovered in some way, because they were still there, apparently, in the 1950s.

The drowning was talked of in hushed tones for months. All these years later, I can still picture the little fair-haired, fairy-like child.

Such a tragedy!

Things That Go Bump

It seems odd that I do not remember the first sirens or the first bombs of the Second World War. At some stage, it was all just there. I would lie in bed and hear the siren go. The sound was exciting, and frightening, too. I was not allowed to get up and get ready to go to the shelter; I had to wait for Mum to call me.

One night the siren had only just died away when there was a huge bang: the house shook, the windows rattled and even my bed seemed to wriggle. I was terrified, but, even so, I did not dare to run downstairs or even to get out of bed. I lay shivering with fear until I heard Mum on the stairs, shouting at me to 'get up and bring your dressing gown'. I grabbed Ted, and my slippers and dressing gown, and rushed onto the landing, and we ran down to the shelter. There were more thumps and gunfire but nothing quite as loud as the first. I felt better in the shelter.

A huge bomb had fallen just on the opposite side of the river, missing three houses and landing in a field. Daddy had seen the explosion from the garden, where he had been fire-watching. It was so loud that it had sounded as though it had fallen in the garden right next to him!

The next day, through Daddy's binoculars, we could just see the hole and a very big pile of earth.

'Why didn't you come straight down when you heard the bang?' asked Daddy next morning.

'I have to wait for Mum to tell me,' I said.

'Mum doesn't mean at times like that.' He seemed amused, but I still didn't know how bad the bangs had to be before I could come down.

The school was higher up in the village, so we could look across the river from the playground and see the big hole much better. We were all standing in a row on the playground wall, gaping at the sheer size of the crater, when a tractor chugged across the field. It stopped, and the man got off to look into the hole. Then he returned to the tractor, collected a package and walked over to sit in the shelter of the hedge to eat his sandwiches.

We could still hear the tractor engine.

'Why hasn't he turned the engine off?' I asked.

A knowledgeable farmer's son spoke up. 'It's the spark plug.'

What was a spark plug?

We all got bored looking at a hole and a chugging tractor and were turning to resume our games when there was an enormous bang. We stared as earth, rocks, smoke and bits of tractor flew up into the air, gradually falling back to the ground with clatters and thumps.

As the smoke cleared, we could see the figure of the man standing by the hedge with his sandwich still in his hand, staring at the pile of metal that a moment ago had been his tractor.

'Cor!' said one of the boys, echoing everyone's thoughts. 'If 'ee 'adent stopped fer 'is dinner, 'eed be a goner!'

This stark possibility destroyed even the boys' excitement—but only for a minute.

The man's lucky escape was the talk of the village for a long time.

'Luckiest man around,' said Daddy. 'The vibration from the tractor probably set the time bomb off.'

Next day, the field was full of army men walking up and down to see if there was any sign that more bombs were buried there. We children were sorry that they did not find any, because we were told that they would have blown them up and that would have been fun to watch.

Pigs, Mice and Puzzles

During my childhood, my father was friendly with a neighbouring farmer named Tom Rayner. There was a funny little unmade-up lane—a secret lane—from the back of the Works fields to his farm. I used to wonder why we sometimes went that way when the proper lane would have been easier.

Well . . . there was a reason. Every time one of his sows farrowed, Tom would fail to declare one piglet to the Ministry of Food.

'A bit dodgy,' said Daddy.

When the piglet had grown big, it was slaughtered, and Tom's various friends would go up the back lane to the farm to be given a joint of pork. The front parlour of the farmhouse had big shutters on the windows, and if ever they were closed, we knew that there was a dead pig hanging from hooks in the ceiling.

The farmer's wife, Edith, used to give me big pieces of cake and mugs (not cups) of tea if I had been allowed to go with my father to collect the pork. I hated to see the pig hanging from the ceiling, but I enjoyed the pork—and the crackling.

Tom and Edith had a little boy called Jim. When scarcely out of nappies, he used to accompany his father everywhere on the farm in the tractor or the trailer. He just went to 'work' when his dad did and came home for meals with him. If he was tired, he'd sleep wherever they happened to be working. He was a wild, happy child, totally devoted to his father.

He started school when I was about eight or nine. He did not understand that he had to sit still or that he could not run out to set off home just when he wanted. He ran round and round the classroom, yelling and lashing out at the teacher, who tried to restrain him. Tom was sent for and removed his son for several months while he gradually made him realise that he had to behave differently in school.

Jim was very bright, but he thought his life with his father would never change. I was sorry for him but at the same time was envious of the life he'd enjoyed before his school days—and which he still enjoyed in the evenings and on weekends.

Whenever we went to the farm, we would see the little curly-haired child in the tractor or plodding along beside his father, fetching the cows in for milking. Perched on a specially made stool, he had been able to milk a cow by hand at the age of four.

One day when I came home from school, Mum was smiling. 'There is a surprise for you in the greenhouse,' she said.

The greenhouse was built onto the back of the house. We kept logs, bits of furniture and tomato plants in it, and against the back wall was the concrete air-raid shelter that Daddy had built.

'Can I—I mean, may I—go and see?'

Normally, shoes had to be cleaned and hands washed before anything else.

'Yes,' said Mum and followed me.

There was a tiny cage on the bench, and four bright little eyes peeped out of the straw.

'Mice! For me?'

Young Jim had brought his mouse into the classroom a week or so before, and it had escaped and caused a lot of fun, and we had all wanted mice from then on.

'Well,' said Mum, 'you went on about Jim's mouse so much that we thought you might like some yourself. But you must look after them: feed them, clean them out, give them water and so on.'

'Oh yes. I will. Thank you.' I was very excited.

Mum seemed as pleased about the mice as she had been about Tig. I was surprised, but I didn't know why.

'It's a boy and girl. What are you going to call them?'

I called the girl mouse Winnie and the boy Bobbie.

When Daddy came in and I had thanked him, I told him what I was calling them.

He burst into laughter. 'I don't know whether Mr. Churchill would be pleased to know that a mouse has been named after him!' I had forgotten that Winston Churchill was called Winnie.

That evening I was allowed to stay up a little later, and I saw Daddy kiss Mum! Apart from a quick 'goodbye' peck, it was the first time I had seen them kiss at all. I went to bed in a sort of hopeful glow. They were nice to each other—and Mum to me—for several days. But then there was a lot of shouting, and Daddy stomped off into the garden and started to dig very quickly. Foolishly, I asked Mum if I might go to help him.

'No,' she snapped. 'Just get off to bed.'

I crept away. It was not even my bedtime.

The nice few days were over, and I wondered why. But at least there was Tig, and I had Winnie and Bobbie now. I cleaned them out regularly, fed and watered them, and stroked their warm little bodies and was rewarded by their obvious excitement when I approached their cage.

Then one day, in their nest of wood shavings, there were four tiny pink naked babies. They were not pretty, but I was thrilled.

These days, a nine- or ten-year-old would know exactly how and why the babies had been created. But even living in the country with animals all around, I did not know about the birds and the bees.

Oddly, I didn't ask about the mice, but one day, as Mum and I were walking through the village, we stopped and Mum talked to a lady. After we moved on, I felt that I could ask a question.

'That lady is going to have a baby, isn't she?'

'Yes, she is. But how did you know?'

'She's got it in her tummy: that's why she's fat. But how does it get out? And how did it get there in the first place?'

Mum went very pink and said, 'We'll talk about that when you are older.'

Later, I heard her say to my father, 'She's starting to ask far too many questions these days.'

But over the next few days it wasn't the questions that were not answered that troubled me, rather the things that I would be told about my mother and my future.

The raids were more frequent now, and seemed to be getting nearer, so we went to bed in the shelter to avoid having to get out of a warm bed to go to a cold one when the siren went. At least I didn't have the problem of guessing how loud the bangs had to be before I could go downstairs.

One evening, Daddy came into the shelter after I had gone to bed and spoke to me very sternly. I had obviously displeased Mum in some way.

'You should be grateful to Mum because she is a better mother to you than your own would have been.'

How I hated being told that! Surely it wasn't true. How could he know? Mummy had loved me—Auntie Jinny had said so. I didn't think Mum did. And I had not been afraid of Mummy, as I often was of Mum.

'Yes, Daddy,' I replied. But I didn't like Daddy for a long time after that, and it was at about this time that I started to call him 'Dad'.

But there was worse to come.

The Country Nurse Remembers

The next morning, Mum said, 'Daddy had a word with you, I believe. Just you remember what he said.'

'Yes, Mum.'

She looked at me in a funny way and said, 'Of course, your mother and father never wanted you in the first place. Grandfather Radford told them to have a child to cement their marriage.' She paused. 'No. They didn't want you at all.'

She went back to the cooking, saying over her shoulder, 'Have you finished cleaning the bedrooms yet?'

'No, Mum.'

'Well, it's high time you had. You know, if you don't buck your ideas up, no one will want you when you grow up, either.'

I crept away to finish sweeping, mopping and dusting the bedrooms, hoping that she would not see my tears.

So, did no one want me?

Mum obviously didn't. Aunt Doris hadn't. Grandmother Radford didn't seem to have. Aunt Lizzy was too busy. And now, it seemed, my mummy and daddy hadn't wanted me in the first place.

What had I done that no one wanted me? Or that no one ever would if I didn't 'buck my ideas up'. What did that mean?

I wasn't really bad, I thought. I didn't get any bad school reports. But I didn't always clean my shoes very well and I was slow at peeling potatoes and I sometimes mumbled instead of speaking up. I hurried home from school, but I must have dawdled now and then because I was a bit late sometimes. I didn't always use toothpaste because some sorts made me feel sick, but I couldn't remember anything else, although there must have been lots of things, I supposed.

But Mummy must have wanted babies because she had another one after me: the baby sister who had died. She wouldn't have done that if she had not liked me, I reasoned, in my innocent, childish, uncomprehending way.

But it didn't seem to help, so I came back to thinking that it must have been my fault. But how could it be my fault *before* I was born?

I don't think I felt anything at all for a long time after that. There did not seem to be anything in me left to hurt, so I didn't feel, didn't think and didn't cry anymore. I suppose it was because I was feeling so miserable that I looked back to the good times; this gave me a warm feeling inside because it was where I believed my heart to be. It must be there in my chest, I reasoned, because that was where I felt the pain when I was in trouble or Mum told me things I didn't want to hear—like not being wanted. And it was where it hurt when I wondered what had happened to Crib.

And that was where I had a warm feeling when I thought about Mummy.

But even thinking about that time could sometimes make me sad, because it was now so long ago and I couldn't get back there because Mummy was dead, and no matter how much I wanted her she would stay dead.

I sometimes talked to her as though she were still alive, mostly just in my head but sometimes out loud when no one was about. But did she hear up there with Jesus? What did people do all day when they had gone to see Jesus? The vicar talked about 'eternal rest', but then we sang about 'rejoicing with the angels'. Some of the gravestones in the churchyard said, 'Asleep in the arms of Jesus,' or 'Fell asleep in the love of God.'

So which was it? Was Mummy asleep? If so, how could Auntie Jinny be so certain that Mummy knew how I was getting on? Or was she chatting with Jesus and the angels?

When I talked to her, did she hear me? And did she answer? I couldn't hear her voice. I would have to ask Auntie Jinny when we next visited.

Make Do and Mend

Life in the 1930s and '40s was very much a 'make do and mend' affair for ordinary people like ourselves. That was the catchword. When the war came, it was even more necessary, as so many ordinary domestic things became unobtainable. Merchant vessels, bringing goods from other countries, were being sunk by U-boats, so the markets and shops were often nearly empty. I'm not sure if I was aware of this at the time or if I learned about it later.

DIY was not a catchphrase, however; it was already a way of life. In fact, I don't think the acronym had been invented. I know Grandpa mended the family shoes on a last in his shed. He mended chairs or beds or anything that was broken. Daddy mended kettles and saucepans when the gas burner had made the bottoms so thin that they leaked. Old saucepans and frying pans were scrubbed with sand when we couldn't get Vim anymore.

I remember once that we had some fun when Daddy was mending a metal teapot. The handle had come off, and he had been riveting it back on. He had just finished when the spout, by which he had been holding the pot, fell off, too. He burst into laughter, threw his hands in the air in mock despair and jumped on the teapot, squashing it flat. I liked that: Daddy being silly did not happen very often these days.

We had tea out of the best china teapot after that. Of course, there were no teabags then, so the loose tea was put in the teapot, and people had tea strainers. Tea out of mugs was almost unheard of. In fact, I don't think china mugs were around at all, only tin ones for men to take to work.

Mum darned socks, let my dresses down, unpicked some of Daddy's old pullovers to save the good wool for a jumper for me or gloves for him. Old curtains were made into clothes, and men's collars and cuffs were turned to hide the frayed bits. This sort of thing had been done for years by careful housewives, but now because of the shortages everyone had to do it.

Rag-rugs, for in front of the fire, were made by cutting up old lisle stockings—tights had not arrived on the scene at that time. Large rugs were turned to even the wear, and old lino was patched or turned round so that the worn bit was under a piece of furniture. Men's trousers were remade to fit a growing son, while knickers were worn back to front when the seat had worn thin.

Clothing coupons did not go far, although growing children were issued with more than grown-ups. New clothes were expensive, anyway, and often they were not available at all because cotton was not getting through from the cotton-growing countries and wool seemed to be in short supply. There were no synthetic fabrics; those came later. So, many of the growing children wore clothes that were far too short in arm and leg or perhaps too big because they had been made to allow for growth. Buttons were removed from defunct clothes and hoarded like gold for shirts and trousers.

Food was not too much of a problem for us, as Dad grew vegetables and soft fruit in the garden; we had the apple orchard, and there were many plum trees beside the private road leading to the Works. In the season, we had plenty, but, without electricity, there was no freezer (very few people had freezers anyway), so the old-fashioned ways of preserving were used.

The Country Nurse Remembers

Potatoes were stored in clamps; apples were wrapped in newspaper and placed in a dark loft, while plums and damsons became jam, and tomatoes were made into chutney. Peas, beans and carrots had to be eaten up, as no way had been found to preserve these, while sprouts, swedes and cabbages seemed to last in the ground for most of the winter. Swedes in particular seemed to be eternal and indestructible, and I remember eating plates full of them. How I hated swedes! Potatoes were never rationed, though, and in fact the general shortages were worse for a few years after the war than during the hostilities.

During the war years, we rarely saw oranges, lemons or bananas, as these were imported. When bananas did get through, some were kept back for small children with Coeliac disease, and we were encouraged to give up our ration, too. I was more than happy to give mine up, as bananas made me very sick!

Meat, fish, sugar, butter, milk, sweets, chocolate, eggs, tinned foods, salt, soap (detergents had not arrived then) and many, many more commodities were rationed (I believe meat and chocolate were still rationed well into the 1950s). Women queued for hours at butcher's shops and fruiterers, clutching their ration books, because, in spite of the fairness of rationing, there was not always enough to go round and it was sometimes first come, first served. I often stood with Mum for long periods for very ordinary goods.

Dad decided to get some geese because the eggs were bigger than chickens' eggs. We had kept chickens for years and ate the old ones when they stopped laying. If you kept chickens, you were not supposed to get the egg ration of one egg a week. I'm not sure how this was policed, if at all, however. A goose, meanwhile, made several good meals. Like most country men, Dad also shot rabbits for the pot. Some men shot pigeons, but Dad said that the amount of meat on them was not worth the effort.

Most housewives baked puddings, pies, cakes and sometimes bread in the 1930s and '40s, but when the war came, ingredients were difficult to get. However, glucose in big yellow tins needed fewer coupons than sugar, while dried eggs were possibly unrationed. Recipes were published for 'eggless cakes', 'sugarless puddings' and 'dried egg omelette'.

People living in cities, with no access to ground for growing vegetables and no hope of keeping chickens or shooting rabbits, were sometimes hungry. But the generally austere diet meant that everyone was a lot slimmer and, in many ways, healthier than they are now, in the twenty-first century. However, the unbalanced diet and the pall of smoke which hung over the industrial cities caused many children to have rickets. Today, we would call this smoke 'smog', but it didn't adopt that name until the 1950s.

Coal, by which most homes were heated, was also by then in short supply. Power stations were coal-fired, and the huge factories making guns, bombs, tanks, aircraft and ammunition needed vast quantities to feed their furnaces. So domestic needs were well down on the list of priorities. People raided woods and forests, chopped down garden trees, burnt rubbish: anything to keep warm.

Again, we were lucky, as there were plenty of gnarled old trees on the Works that could be felled and chopped up. The remaining 'chaps' brought their wheelbarrows and took logs home with them. Once more, people in the cities were worse off than us; centres were opened where old people could gather to keep warm and drink the soup on offer. Many were trying to survive on the old-age pension, which was meagre and insufficient to meet the inflated prices of necessities.

Other things in short supply included ink, paper, pencils, books, flashlight batteries, petrol, paraffin, needles, nails and screws. I remember having to write lessons on the back of rolls of wallpaper that Governess found in her loft because the exercise books had not arrived.

At about this time, Dad, at last, decided that I should stay up on Fridays and Saturdays to hear the six o'clock news, as he felt that I should know what was going on in the world. So I began to understand a bit more about the progress of the war. I remember the deep voice of Alvar Lidell, saying, 'London calling'; then there were the lighter tones of Stuart Hibberd and the gravelly ones of Bruce Belfrage, telling us of victories and defeats in about equal measure, as it seemed to me.

I was excited to hear Bruce Belfrage, because, in 1940, during the London bombing, he had been reading the news when Broadcasting House took a direct hit. People listening heard the explosion—it was so loud—but Bruce Belfrage went on reading as though nothing had happened, although he was covered in soot and plaster and had had to brush the dirt off his notes. I asked Dad about it.

'It was to keep up morale,' said Dad, who had been most impressed by the cool-headed announcer.

I supposed that 'morale' meant cheerfulness.

It seemed to be in short supply. Like everything else.

The Bath Blitz

At the Thursday school church service, the vicar had said that we must be stalwart. We had no idea what that meant, so we all nodded and tried to look as though we did. Then he said that we must have faith. We had lots of that because we knew, without a shadow of a doubt, that God was on our side. Everyone said so.

But over several nights in April 1942, God seemed to have forgotten about Bath. Bath was being bombed out of existence, said Dad. How could that happen? Bath was the only town I knew, but it was too big to be bombed out of existence, surely.

The thumps and explosions and the gunfire had been getting closer over the previous few nights as Bristol was getting it. The factories, docks and airfields were the main targets, but houses were bombed too, and many people were killed. The noise of the attacks on Bristol was frightening, but it went on for so many nights that I eventually slept through most of it.

On this particular night, however, the noise was even louder, and the bombs seemed nearer. The shelter shook, and I could hear the tinkling of glass as parts of the greenhouse shattered. I could see the glow of the fires caused by the incendiary bombs that were raining down on the village and the fields around us. This was much worse than before. I was told not to undress but just to lie in my bunk with all my clothes on. Tig was in the shelter with us and kept whining. He did not like the thumps and bangs. Dad kept popping in and out of the shelter. He was fire-watching because the Works was in danger from the incendiaries. He and Mr. Burn, the foreman, took it in turns, one watching one night and the other the next. But on this night they were both watching together because there were so many bombs. When Dad appeared on one occasion, his clothes were muddy from where he had flung himself onto the ground as a particularly close bomb had sent showers of mud and shrapnel into the air.

'Bath's getting it again tonight,' said Daddy. 'I can't see why Bath. There's nothing there for them.'

At the time, these raids on Bath were a mystery to people, as there were virtually no factories—and certainly no airfield or docks—in the city. The mainline railway came through Bath and went on to Bristol and the West, but that did not seem enough reason for the vicious attack.

After the war ended, however, we heard these were called Baedeker raids, but none of us knew anything about that at the time. (In 1937, a German called Baedeker had written a guide to historical and cultural British towns and cities, such as York, Exeter and Bath, and the Germans used this information to identify and bomb such places. Bath had beautiful Georgian buildings, and many of these were destroyed. I remember the piles of rubble.)

Dad was worried because all the pipes coming to the Works were from Bath and its surrounds, and he knew that there would be a lot of damage to them.

Mum sat quietly knitting by the light of the oil lamp to keep her mind off it. She was very worried, because her parents lived in Bath and there was no way of knowing if they were being bombed; her cousin, Harry, was a patient in the Mineral Water

Hospital in the centre of Bath, too. Dad was not very hopeful about Harry's chances. But all they could do was wait until morning and hope for the best.

'Hope for the best' was on everyone's lips.

The best of what?, I wondered.

Bath was behind a hill as you looked out from Meadow View but was only about three miles away as the crow flies, so we could see the angry red sky and the clouds of orange smoke. The searchlights continuously swept the sky, occasionally picking out a plane, and then the guns would start their 'crump-crump' sound. How did they know the plane was one of 'theirs'—it was so high up? Occasionally they must have shot one, because we heard the whine of the engines getting closer and closer as the aircraft plunged to the ground. It always sounded as though it were going to hit us, but none did. There was nothing we could do, anyway, but just cower in the shelter and 'hope for the best'. Most of the planes crashed in fields and woods, often catching fire and adding their own red and orange light and black smoke clouds to the chaos in the sky.

The noise of bombs and guns went on and on until the sky began to lighten towards morning. Then we heard the drone of many planes over the house and the village. Dad explained they were making for home in France or Germany—usually France, where the Germans had built airfields, because Germany was much farther away and the planes could not carry enough fuel to fly so far.

'I hope they land in the Channel,' said Dad. But many of them crashed in the villages around, often killing people on the ground. I think I dozed off, but I don't think Dad and Mum slept at all that night.

I did not go to school the next day—I don't believe anyone knew if the school was still there. So I was at home when the telephone calls started. We were amazed to find that the phone lines were still working.

Dad went rushing off to Bath.

'Find out what you can about my mum and dad,' called Mum, as he disappeared.

Dad had to go to the worst-affected areas to inspect any water and drainage pipes that had been blown up. Gas pipes were leaking and the gasometer at the gasworks had been hit, so the gas supply was cut off to hundreds of homes, including ours.

Dad told us later that the city was still burning and in utter chaos, with people being dug out of collapsed buildings, huge craters appearing everywhere, roads being blocked or cordoned off and unexploded bombs being made safe by the bomb-disposal chaps.

'I wouldn't have their job for all the tea in China,' Dad had said. 'It's very dangerous work.'

But he had to go in amongst all the devastation and near these bombs to inspect the various pipes and recommend the action to be taken in repairing them. So he was in danger, too.

Later in the day, he found Grandma and Granddad S.—Mum's parents. They were in a neighbour's house because their own had been so badly shattered by the blast from a bomb in the road that it was unsafe. Dad brought them home to Meadow View.

Grandma S. was hysterical and couldn't stop sobbing, while Granddad S. was 'stoic', Mum said. I had heard that word before and thought it must mean 'silent', because he seemed unable to say anything at all for a long time. He just stood and stared out of the window.

Before Daddy could eat his lunch, another telephone call came to say that the Mineral Water Hospital had been so badly hit that it was just a pile of rubble. The patients had been evacuated in time and they were all safe, but there was nowhere for them to go.

Mum's cousin Harry came from Southsea, which was a long way off, so he had given her name as a contact. Dad set off for Bath to collect him.

Harry had a condition that made his back completely stiff in the upright position so that he could not sit, so in order for Dad to get him home, he had to take the passenger seat out of the car and help Harry onto the back seat, with his legs stretched out in front of him so that he was almost lying down.

Suddenly our house was full. I was very sorry for Grandma and Granddad S. because their house was in ruins—or so we thought at the time. It was not quite as bad as that, and later they managed to rescue some furniture, which went into storage until after the war. I was even sorrier for Harry, though he was quite cheerful. He said he was glad to be alive and he hadn't had any possessions with him to lose.

Mum ran about arranging the spare bedroom for Grandma and Granddad S., and Dad got a bed from somewhere and put it in the other room for Harry, as he could not go upstairs. We had a downstairs lavatory, but I don't recall where Harry washed; perhaps a bowl in the other room.

I was able to fetch and carry and run about helping, which I enjoyed. This was something real; not just the usual bedroom- or stair-cleaning. I even managed to cheer Grandma up a bit by brushing her hair and finding her perfume in her handbag. I helped Mum make up the bed for Harry and arrange the furniture so that he could get around with his two sticks. He was always singing or humming. And he talked to me about all sorts of things: my school friends, my books, his house in Southsea, the weird treatments that he was getting for his back . . . Other grown-ups wanted to know what I was doing at school but once I had told them never seemed to know what else to say.

With the gas cut off, Mum had to cook on the old Rayburn-type range, which she had not used before, but she made things like stews and mince with heaps of vegetables and bottled fruit with custard. Catering for the sudden influx of people must have been very difficult, as our rations had to stretch until our visitors could get their new ration books. The old ones were somewhere in the ruins of their homes.

Mum must have been exhausted, but she seemed to be in a good mood as she hurried around. Dad looked grey with tiredness and the worry of the pipes in Bath, but Grandma was the only one who showed how upset everyone must have been feeling inside. I know that I enjoyed having lots of people around and being needed instead of being sent off to bed early.

The following night it was just as noisy. The planes could be heard approaching before it was properly dark.

'They are early tonight. There won't be anything left in Bath at this rate,' said Daddy, but he was so tired that he fell asleep in the fireside armchair.

Normally we would all have gone to the shelter, but Mum said to leave him. She tried to get Grandma into the shelter, but she refused, saying that she would not be able to breathe in there and she would take her chances in the house. She wouldn't let Granddad leave her either, and Harry could not get there at all. So Mum decided to stay with them, and I was the only one in the shelter.

I hated it. The bombs and guns seemed much worse when I was alone. I think it was Harry who suggested that Tig should join me. That was a bit better, but he was too frightened and barked to be let back into the house. Eventually, Dad woke.

'Where's Julia?' he asked.

'In the shelter,' said Mum.

'All by herself? That's not right, Mildred. The child will be terrified. I'll go and lie on my bunk.'

So Dad came into the shelter, lay down and, in spite of the fearful noise, was instantly asleep. That was better, but Mum was not pleased.

Life at Meadow View was quite chaotic with so many people living there, but I enjoyed the company, especially Harry's.

There was no school the next day, but I don't recall whether it was because it was a day off anyway or because it had been decided to keep the building closed. I know that some of the windows had been shattered either by the blast from bombs in nearby fields or the shockwaves of the roaring guns. It was an old granite building, and bits of mortar had been dislodged by the Bristol raids; now the Bath raids were causing more and more to fall out.

The coal had not arrived for the boiler either, but I don't think we would have had the heating on in April anyway. There was one big fat radiator in each of the two classrooms, and these were fed from the coal-fired boiler. The boiler man came in every morning before school to clear out and stoke the furnace. Sometimes he was late and the fire had gone out altogether, and then he would say some bad words and growl a lot, so we kept well away from him. On these mornings, it would be dinnertime before the rooms warmed up.

The boiler was located in a dark passageway near the girls' lavatories, thus ensuring that those facilities stayed frost-free in winter. The boys' lavatories were outside in the playground and froze up, so that they could not be used until the thaw came—which meant the boys had to use the girls' lavatories. We hated this, of course, because as far as we were concerned, boys were dirty and made the floor wet and didn't pull the chain or wash their hands. They jeered at any girls they happened to meet on the way in or out. The girls always complained to Governess, who wrinkled her nose and stalked off to the lavatories, her high heels clicking threateningly on the stone floors. She muttered in disgust at the mess and sent for the boiler man to clean up. He did some more grumbling and growling and Governess kept all the boys in after school. But it was all just as bad the next winter.

The Country Nurse Remembers

I remember a lady in an overall cleaned the classrooms. There was no vacuum cleaner, so she swept the old boards—which seemed to produce more and more dust, the more she swept. Sometimes she brought a handful of wet, used tea leaves which she scattered over the floor before sweeping. Curious, we asked her why.

'Don't you girls know nothin'?' she replied. 'These be to lay the dust. Gawd knows what yous lot'll do when yous grows up.' (Luckily, 'Gawd' had given us vacuum cleaners by then.)

The overall lady flicked a duster about as well, and Governess tutted a lot because her desk was always covered in chalk dust.

Dad had rushed off to Bath again early the next morning and came home for lunch. I heard the car and wanted to go to greet him, but I was dusting and tidying the other room, which was now referred to as 'Harry's room', while Harry was stomping to the door to go into the hall. He had reached the doorway but was so slow that I ran out of the other door, into the greenhouse, out into the yard, in the back door, through the kitchen and dining room and into the hall to say 'Hello' to Dad while poor Harry was still getting through the door.

Harry was singing. It was one of the war songs, and when Dad heard it he joined in, as I did, and we all sang together: 'Pack up your troubles in your old kit bag'.

Harry, who was never going to get better, was an inspiration to us all, said Dad.

When Mum heard us, she just shouted, 'What a row!'

I was allowed to eat with everyone else now because it was easier for Mum to serve us all together. I seemed to be getting a little more food, too. Granddad S. had some very strong views about the Germans, the British Army, the Ministry, the War Office, Mr. Churchill and just about everything else, and he thumped the table to emphasise his points. Mum thought he'd break the crockery, but Dad just smiled and wagged his head.

I thought it was all good fun. In spite of Dad's worries, Mum's short temper (not always directed at me, now), Grandma S.'s hysterics and Granddad S.'s funny views, I liked these meals. Although not allowed to speak, I felt part of what was going on rather than being told to get along, get out of the way, as before.

After we had finished, I always did the washing up. Harry insisted on drying up. So long as he could remain standing and leaning on something, he was able to help. So he dried and piled the dishes up until they looked precarious, and then he'd stop and I would put them away. Then we'd start again. There was something real and necessary about this work, and Mum had too much to do to time me doing things. Harry was such fun!

Busy Times at Meadow View

The next night was much quieter. The Germans had got fed up with Bath, now they'd nearly finished it off, Dad said.

We heard the thump of a distant bomb now and then, and the guns went crump-crump when the search lights, endlessly sweeping the sky, picked out an enemy plane, but Dad and Mum and I were able to have a much-needed sleep in the shelter without the worry of the bombing being too close. I don't know if Grandma S. and Granddad S. stayed in their bed or came downstairs. Harry claimed that he slept through 'anything and everything', but I think he must have been in a lot of pain, because the pills by his bed were always gone in the morning.

Dad was at the Works 'catching up' the next day but went into Bath again in the afternoon, taking Granddad S. with him to see if they could arrange for some furniture to be rescued from the house and put into storage. Granddad's piano, a smart modern one, was dusty but in one piece.

'Will need tuning,' he grumbled.

Somehow, they found someone to bring it to Meadow View. There, it went into the other room, joining our own piano— much older and larger—Harry's bed and chair and bedside table, two armchairs and a settee. It was a very big room!

Granddad was an organist and pianist, and he played every day. Grandma said that he thumped so hard that it made her head hurt. Mum said, 'Phooee.' Granddad had been far enough into Bath with Dad to see the burnt-out shell of the church where he played the organ. He was very upset, but Dad said it was better that than people's homes. That church was never rebuilt.

On Dad's way into Bath, two ladies, walking along the road, had asked for a lift by waggling their thumbs, like the soldiers on leave did. Dad had picked them up, thinking that they were Bath people going back to get things from their ruined homes, like Granddad. He chatted with them and asked if this was the case.

'Oh, no,' they said. 'We don't live there. We just want to look at all the damage.'

Dad was furious. He stopped the car and ordered them out.

'People like that are just sightseers,' he raged, when he came home. 'They are glorying in other people's misery and just cluttering the place up. The authorities have enough to deal with. They ought to be shot! Everyone is trying to get things moving again, and they don't need idiots like that around the place!'

Dad rumbled on and on until Mum told him to eat his tea. But more exciting and unbelievable was his next tale, which he told us after he had eaten his tea.

In one of the areas worst hit, the bomb-disposal men had located an unexploded bomb almost buried under the remains of a large building. Dad had to assess the damage to the pipes going to and from this building, and he got out of there as soon as he could, he said. But the disposal men had dug around the huge bomb, shoring up the muddy walls of the crater with boards. It was dinnertime when Dad was there, and he couldn't believe his eyes when he saw 'those two fools' sitting on the bomb to eat their sandwiches! Later, when they were told off by whoever was in charge, they said that they were pretty sure that, doing the job that they did, they were going to get blown up at some time, so why worry. I thought that was very sad. Dad said that they had a death wish.

After the war, we heard that many of the crews of the fighters and bombers felt the same. They said it was the only way to cope. I tried to imagine how that would feel, but I couldn't.

Gradually, more and more of Grandma's clothes arrived at Meadow View. Mum said she had far too many, and where were we going to put them all? The big wardrobe on the landing was filled, and still there were more posh coats and feathery dresses and sparkly jackets, so some things were hung on the back of my bedroom door.

Among these was a fox-fur. It was a fur cape that ladies wore around their shoulders over a coat or jacket. It had a long 'body', with a tail and a head with glass eyes. This was horrid. The eyes caught any ray of light and were quite frightening in the night, as they seemed to stare at me in my bed.

I don't remember why I was sleeping in my bedroom again instead of the shelter. The sirens still went almost nightly, and bombs and guns could be heard until daybreak, so why we were back in the house I do no know. I have always thought that we spent about a year sleeping in the shelter—or it certainly felt like it.

In the end I found the courage to ask Mum if the fox-fur could go somewhere else, but she just told me not to be silly. Harry was there, however, and winked at me behind Mum's back. When I went to bed, the fox had gone.

Harry seemed to be on my side. Granddad said very little, Grandma sometimes told me to do things in a way that I knew Mum would not like, and that was awkward, but Harry watched and listened and understood how things were.

'Try to stick up for yourself a bit more,' he said to me.

But I didn't.

Animals

During the early years of the war, Dad decided to get a cow so that we would have milk and possibly meat, if she had a calf. Everyone thought that food might get very scarce; in fact, starvation on a massive scale was deemed possible. People would be eating rats and cats, it was said, and—horrifyingly—dogs.

'But we wouldn't eat Tig,' I stated with confidence, as we discussed these issues.

'Yes, we would,' said Dad. 'If we had to.'

'We wouldn't! No, we wouldn't!' I forgot that I was not supposed to argue. I felt sick!

'Only if we were starving. Really starving,' replied Dad. He seemed to understand.

'No, no, no . . . ,' I went on screaming, but only in my head. I was outwardly in control again, but inwardly I was horrified. I could not get this awful possibility out of my mind. It just would not happen! Poor Tig had more cuddles over the next few days than even *he* knew how to cope with.

The cow was a Friesian—black and white and huge. Friesians are apparently good milkers. We must have given her a name, but I cannot recall what it was. I had very little to do with her. In common with many girls at that time, my role was almost exclusively domestic (except for weeding), and I was kept busy indoors—much, much busier than any of my school friends. On the occasions when I *was* allowed to help outside, I was very happy. All my life I have preferred outside work. Given the things I enjoyed doing the most, I often used to think that I should have been born a boy!

I was certainly involved in the making of butter, however. Dad turned what had been a coal-house into the dairy. It took a lot of cleaning and a lot of paint! We had big round pans about six inches deep, into which the warm milk was poured. It was allowed to settle for a short while, and then I had to skim off the cream, which was thick and yellow. I had a sort of metal saucer with which to do this. If you dipped it in too deeply, you got milk mixed with the cream, and then the butter would not 'turn'. The cream was put in a big jar called a 'churn', which had a wooden lid with a handle on the outside and paddles attached to the inside. You patiently turned the handle, sometimes for hours, so that the paddles swished through the cream, gradually making it thicken and eventually turning it to butter. It was a boring job in a way, but I liked doing it: I would be churning away in the dining room, with Dad and Mum, rather than in the other room by myself.

I think we had the cow for about two years; she didn't have a calf, and her milk eventually dried up. By then Dad and Mum were a bit fed up because there was usually too *much* milk—even making some into butter didn't use it all up.

'Not worth all the work,' said Dad.

Then Dad thought that it would be good to have pigs. They could live on scraps from our kitchen and those of our neighbour; they would not have to be milked and should have lots of piglets—ensuring a good meat supply if things got bad. So an enormous and very bad-tempered sow arrived. I like pigs, but she was quite scary, and I was glad to keep away from her.

She was due to farrow on a particular date, and Dad said that he would stay up all that night with her to see that nothing went wrong. Several weeks went by, and then, one morning, I heard a lot of shouting. When I came downstairs to go to school, Dad was sitting holding one pink little pig and trying to spoon some milk into its mouth.

'I got the date wrong,' said Dad, sadly. 'Well, it was the right date, but she had them the night *before*, not the night *of* . . . She has killed the lot except this little chap. He rolled under the bars, and she couldn't reach him. She bit their heads off as they were born.' Dad called her a few bad names then . . . at least I think they were bad names. I was so sorry for all the little dead piglets.

I asked what would happen to this one. Evidently, Dad was going to the chemist to get a baby's bottle to try to keep the little pink scrap alive.

So we brought the little fellow up on the bottle. And because of the funny noises he made, we called him 'Chuggy'. He was very demanding and needed feeding every few hours. Tig was intrigued and watched Chuggy when he tried to run about; Chuggy seemed to think that Tig was his mother, following the dog everywhere. This was a good thing, because although Chuggy was kept in the house (for warmth and convenience for feeding), he didn't make any mess. He would potter to the back door with Tig when Tig wanted to go out, and he would follow him, presumably watching and understanding that he was 'spending a penny or tuppence', and copy him. No one believed that a little pig could train himself in this way, but that was what happened, and, after the first few days, we had no puddles or mess at all. He was very clean and pink; not at all smelly, as people think pigs can be.

Tig and pig ran around playing together, barking and grunting and knocking each other over, and, for a few weeks, they had good fun. One morning I was allowed to take Tiggy for a walk down the private road towards the Works. Chuggy objected to being parted from him and started to make a terrible noise in protest, so I asked if I could take him, as well. All was well for a few yards, and then Chuggy got homesick and ran all the way home, squealing with terror, while Tig had run off in the other direction. I eventually caught Tig, and when we got home, there was Chuggy on the back doorstep, patiently waiting to go in.

But a pig grows very quickly and Chuggy was soon big and heavy, and Tig became frightened of him. He would also butt the backs of our legs with his hard snout. This was not comfortable. He was off the bottle now but still tried to get onto our laps expecting his milk, as he had before.

One evening, he was running around in the other room and decided to rub himself against the back of the settee, which was traditionally placed in front of the fire. He pushed so hard that the settee moved swiftly forwards, ending up in the hearth. Thankfully Mum saw what happened, or we would have had a burnt settee—or worse, perhaps. He had to go!

Dad built a pigsty in the lean-to greenhouse. We left the windows open for air, but he was quite warm . . . just very cross at being turned out of the house.

He went on growing until he was enormous. Eventually, we could keep him no longer, and he was sent to the butcher. I was very upset, as I had become fond of him. Dad had decided that pigs were not easy, so the sow went, too. I was not so very sorry to see her go and was glad that she took her bad temper with her!

Petrol rationing was getting severe, and often there was none even for folk like Dad, who had an allowance for work trips. Private outings had stopped altogether. So the next animal to arrive was a pony. Again, surprisingly, I do not remember his name. A beautiful, well-sprung carriage came with him. It was very smart and comfortable and had a coat-of-arms painted on the side. I was most impressed, but I never did find out whose arms they were or why the carriage was sold to us with the emblem still on the side.

Dad was not very good at handling the pony. He was used to Punch and Charlie, the Shires, who were so placid and always seemed to know what to do without being told. The pony was probably young; he was certainly very frisky.

Mr. Burn, the foreman, was experienced in handling horses and tried to teach Dad how different a pony was from a car. 'You got to remember, Boss, as how this 'ere 'orse 'as a leg at each corner instead of four wheels and ee 'as 'is own idears 'bout where 'ees goin'. Them reins aint a steerin' wheel!'

Mum and I laughed at Dad's efforts, but Mum was too frightened to go in the carriage. (We called it a 'trap', which was a shame, because it was far too posh to be a trap.)

I had a few rides up and down the road to the Works, while Dad practised with the reins and the commands. I thought he was very clever to learn so fast. I liked bowling along in the fresh air with the pony clip-clopping in front.

But one day when Dad took him out onto the lane, it ended in disaster. No one knew that the pony had a dislike of manhole covers. Perhaps it was the clank that his hooves made on the metal. So, Dad was happily relaxing with the reins held lightly in his hands when, to avoid a manhole cover, the pony suddenly side-stepped—straight into the path of one of the very few vehicles still on the roads. A big lorry!

The lorry stopped in time, but the pony was frightened by the screech of the brakes and took off at a gallop. Dad just held on and pulled the reins, but the carriage was swaying from side to side and bumping about very close to the river. They were almost into the village before Dad gradually brought the terrified pony under control. By then, he was shaking with shock and the effort of hauling on the reins. He walked 'that wretched horse' home, and that was that! The pony had to go.

The Country Nurse Remembers

With the Bath Blitz in the past, and the house full of people, Dad's mind turned to food again.

One dark, rainy Saturday evening, I was told that Dad, Mum and I were going in the car to pick something up from a farm. I was intrigued and excited to be included in the adventure.

The farm was not an ordinary farm. There were no cows or sheep but lots of goats. Goat farms were unheard of: nobody drank goat's milk or ate goat meat. After a lot of talking and laughing, we went out to a stall where there were two goats, a mother goat with a baby. The nanny goat was grey with kind eyes and a beard and was quite happy for us to stroke her. The baby was about the size of a small dog, rather fluffy and very pretty.

I realised that this was to be the next venture.

'Have they got names?' I asked.

'Oh,' said the farmer. 'Babbie were born in the Bath Blitz. Us was in the shelter and knowed nothin' about it. In the mornin' there 'er were. So us called Babbie "Blitz". Big un is "Nan". 'Er's a good milker and Blitz is near weaned. You like 'em, young lady?'

'Oh yes, I do,' I replied. I had never been called 'young lady' before. I felt quite grown-up.

''Ow be you getting them back, then?' The nice man looked doubtfully at the Ford Eight.

'Julia will sit on my wife's knee; we'll fold the rear seats down and put the goats in the back.'

The man scratched his head. 'Aint never 'eard o' goats sittin' in the back seat of a car, afore.' He roared with laughter.

But that is exactly what we did. The goats took some persuading to get into the back of the car but, once there, seemed quite happy. Nan snorted down the back of my neck all the way home, while Blitz tried to eat my hair.

Dad had made a sort of stall for them for night-time, but they would be out in the paddock during the day. They trotted into their straw bed, were given drinks and some nuts to eat and we left them alone to settle down.

Nan was, indeed, a good milker; goats do not give as much milk as cows, so we did not have the same problem we'd had with the cow. I do not remember making butter either, but perhaps we did. I do remember hating the taste of goat's milk. But, of course, I could not say so, and I had to drink it.

Goat's milk and cheese is very healthy and fashionable now, but at the time we were considered to be most odd.

Gradually, we acquired more goats, including a billy goat, who became daddy to Nan's twins, born the next year. He was very wild and always escaping from his field, and Dad got very cross with him. I was told not to give the goats names because we would be eating them at some point. When the twins were young, I tried not to think of having to eat them one day; they were so sweet.

As it happened, we did not eat them. But for a very sad reason: they fell into one of the big tanks of water on the Works and were drowned.

Grandma and Granddad S. were still living with us when we once tried goat meat for Sunday dinner. Mum had told Grandma that it was chicken because she knew that Grandma would refuse to eat goat. Grandma did not guess, but Granddad, who did not approve of lies—even white ones—told her after dinner. From then on, she would not even eat *chicken* in case it was goat. So the white lie did more harm than good, as Granddad said, severely.

We kept the goats until after the end of the war. Food became shorter and shorter in supply than ever then, and Dad said he was glad we had them.

So was I.

Tig was safe as long as we had goats.

Train to Auntie Jinny

Harry left us to go home to Southsea. I was sorry to lose a friend; an ally. Some suitable transport had been found for his return; he had friends there to help him, District Nurses to care for him and a flat that had been adapted to suit his needs. Harry's bed was taken back to wherever it had come from, the other room was rearranged and it was as if Harry had never been there.

Grandma and Granddad S.'s house would not be rebuilt until after the war was over, they were told. Grandma could not understand that everyone was too busy just trying to survive to bother about them, as they had a roof over their heads. Many people were being housed in halls, churches and derelict buildings. Granddad was earnestly following the progress of the war and paid little attention to her complaints. As an ex-serviceman, his main interest was listening to the news and thumping the table, whilst delivering his forceful opinion. Grandma and Mum seemed to have lots of arguments, but I could never work out what they were about.

Occasionally, our vicar would ask Granddad to play the organ for a service in the parish church, as the regular organist had been called up. Granddad was delighted to 'keep his hand in', he said. There was no power to the church, so on Saturdays

I occasionally accompanied him to pump the bellows when he went to practise the hymns for Sunday. I enjoyed being in the lovely old building and listening to the organ, as I pushed the big handle up and down to work the pump. It was hard work, and if I flagged a bit the organ would begin to make weird groaning noises. (Some big man pumped for the actual services.) It is possible that my love of organ music stems from those afternoons.

Granddad played all manner of tunes on his piano in the other room at home: some hymns, some well-known songs and a lot of classical music. I liked it when he played dance tunes. I would leap about and twirl round to the rhythm of the music. Granddad said that I had a good ear—whatever that meant.

One day, he had been playing very serious music for a long time, so I asked if he would play some dance music. 'Good gracious, no, child!' he replied, sounding very severe. 'It's Sunday. We do not have dance music on Sundays.'

At about this time, Grandma had a really big row with Mum and arranged to spend a few days with a friend in Bath. Granddad went with her to catch up with some old friends from his church and to keep the peace, he said.

So Dad decided that we would go to see Auntie Jinny, but it would have to be by train because of the petrol situation. I was quite excited at the thought of a long train journey. Mum and I had been into Bath by train to see Grandma and Granddad before the bombing; but that was only a short distance on the LMS line. The village also had the GWR railway, and each line had a station at that time. Now there is only one line still passing through the village, but there are no stations, so the trains just race through without stopping.

I don't remember which line we travelled on to see Auntie Jinny, but we ended our journey in Cheltenham. To me, the trip itself was an adventure, but more important was seeing Auntie Jinny again. It must have been about two years since our last visit because I was now ten years old.

The cottage, the street and the town seemed just the same. I think Cheltenham had suffered some bombing, but the rest of the Cotswolds were almost untouched, and it was nice to walk around Winchcombe without seeing piles of rubble or big gaps where buildings used to stand. The bombing had more or less stopped in our part of the country, but Bath and Bristol were very sad sights as a result of those terrible raids.

Auntie Jinny was as lovely as ever. She greeted me with a great big hug and held my hand while she said 'Hello' to Dad and Mum.

'You are growing up, little one. We will have some lovely walks together, and you can tell me all that has been happening,' she said.

Auntie was too old to go for long walks, but we went into the town, round the little back lanes and into the churchyard. We had done this before because she always kept 'dear Frank's' grave tidy and put flowers on it in the summer and lovely red leaves in the autumn. We sat on a seat in the sun, near the grave, and chatted.

I told her how ill I had been shortly after our last visit. She was quite shocked, as Dad and Mum had not let her know. I assured her that it was all right, because Mum had been nice to me while I was ill. Auntie looked a bit funny, and I think I heard her say, 'So I should think,' but she spoke so quietly that I was not sure. She clutched my hand very firmly. I was so happy just to be with her.

But there was something I had to ask her.

'Auntie, if I had died and gone to see Jesus, would I have seen Mummy?'

'Of course, you would. She would have been waiting with Jesus. I know I shall see my dear Frank again when I die.' Auntie was totally convinced about such things.

'But, would Mummy know me now? I've got so big that she might not recognise me.' This had been a worry for a while. I had realised that if ever I did get to see Mummy, she would look the same as I remembered. But I was changing—growing—and I would not look like the little girl that she had left. Had not *wanted* to leave, Auntie corrected me. I sometimes wished that the last five or so years had just not happened and that I was still four or five years old and still had Mummy.

'Jesus would make sure that your mummy knew you, little one. But you are not going to die for years and years.'

'They didn't say, but I think I might have nearly died when I was so ill.'

Auntie murmured, 'And they didn't tell me.' She seemed upset, and I suddenly thought that she might say something to Dad and Mum, which might make it look as though I had been complaining.

'Auntie, it's all right. Please don't say anything, will you?'

She looked at me sadly and sighed, shaking her head. Then, taking my hand, she rose and we wandered off, through the trees, back to the road. She told me a little story.

Near the town was the lovely old Sudeley Castle, which we had seen through the trees in the days before the war. But now the grounds were surrounded by barbed wire and big fences, and no one was allowed near. It was a prison camp for Italian soldiers who had been captured by the British. Lots of big huts could be seen, and sometimes the Italian men were walking about between them. I was a bit confused about Italians because they fought on the German side, but later they changed sides and fought *against* the Germans. I couldn't understand this at all. In company with most people, Auntie thought they were just as bad as the Germans and not trustworthy. She did not like the way that the authorities, who did not consider them to be a danger, allowed the prisoners to walk into town.

One day, she had been tending 'dear Frank's' grave as usual, when an Italian prisoner stopped beside her and watched what she was doing. She was a bit nervous at first, but he tried to talk to her in his broken English.

'This your man?'

'Yes, my husband,' said Auntie.

'Very sad. Much long dead?'

'Yes. He was killed in the Great War.' Auntie thought the Italian was very kind to ask about 'dear Frank'.

'You very nice lady . . . talk to prisoner. Sorry . . . your husband.'

And the Italian wandered off.

After that, Auntie changed her mind about *all* the Italians, telling everyone how kind they were, but when she told Dad this tale, he was not so impressed and just said, 'Hmm.'

We did not do anything exciting—you couldn't in the war because of petrol rationing and problems with food. About the only restaurants where you might get a meal if you were out for the day were called 'British Restaurants'. They were not ordinary restaurants: they were run by something called the 'local authority'. But there weren't any near Winchcombe, so we always took sandwiches if we were out at lunchtime.

None of these restrictions bothered me. We were at Auntie Jinny's house, and that was all that mattered.

One evening, we all went to a film being shown at the local hall. There was no cinema for miles. It was terribly cold in the hall, and the film broke down from time to time and an old lady came forward and played tunes on a piano until they got it going again. Although about the war at sea, the film was very funny in parts. There was a ship's cat that seemed to warn the men of an attack and was called 'the intelligent cat'. Auntie had a cat at the time, and we teased her, saying that her cat was not as intelligent as the one in the film. She found this very funny and changed the cat's name to 'Intelligent Cat'. I wondered how she would call it in—it seemed a very long name to shout down the garden.

All too soon, the visit was over, and we went home on the train. I think it was another four years until I saw Auntie Jinny again.

And a lot had changed by then.

The War Effort

Perhaps it was because of all the bombing that the local schools became involved in 'the war effort'. Suddenly, there were all sorts of projects to raise money for people who had been bombed out, and for soldiers and seamen and all manner of other folk.

One morning Governess popped her head into the playground before school and called four girls in to help her. We were told to take some large, bulky parcels into the top classroom.

It was called the 'top' classroom because it was for the older pupils—or the 'big ones'. I was now about ten and so was a member of this class. The little ones were taught in the other classroom by Miss Barnes most of the time. As the wall between the rooms was only a folding wooden screen, there was always a terrific din, said Governess, and when she couldn't stand it any longer, she went in there to 'restore order'.

When the big ones had all assembled, Governess produced lots of huge balls of very thick white wool. Every child in the class had to take several of these home, together with a sheet of paper with a picture of a long seaman's sock, the instructions and some huge knitting needles. The boys handled the wool as though it might bite. They were mortified to be associated with knitting! We were to *tell*—not *ask*—our mothers to knit a pair of these socks, return them to school and then more wool would be issued.

I was very worried. I had never 'told' Mum to do anything—how was I to do this? I made sure that I *ran* most of the way home so that there was not a chance of being late, and I hoped that Grandma S. would be there. It seemed easier to talk to Mum if someone else was present.

I took my bundle in. Mum looked at it and frowned, but before she could say anything I held up the picture of the socks and said, 'Governess says that all the mums have to knit these socks for the seamen and then they have to go back to school and then the mums have to knit some more.' This was all in one breath.

It worked. Mum glanced at Grandma, and then at the wool and pattern, and began to laugh!

'I have never knitted a sock in my life,' she said. 'This wool is so thick, it should knit up quickly, though. Well, I'll do what I can.'

In the end, she liked knitting with this rather greasy wool and the big needles. It all turned into a sort of competition. The mums tried to be the first to finish the initial pair and therefore get more wool for the second. Governess was pleased but was kept very busy sending for more wool. Dad got the idea that if Mum could knit socks for sailors, she could knit socks (the ordinary sort) for him. I think she knitted his socks for the rest of his life.

The 'war effort' that I found fun was the 'Scrap Iron Drive'. One day the local policeman came to the school and explained that in order to make armaments—we guessed that he meant guns and things—the factories needed raw materials. What did he mean by that? 'Raw' to us meant baby carrots or scraped skin! However, he told us that we were to form pairs and go round all the houses in the village asking people for their scrap iron. This could be old pots and pans, old garden implements, garden benches . . . anything that was metal. We called it all 'iron'. This 'drive' was to start on Saturday and continue for several weeks.

When he had gone, Governess paired us off and said that we were to tell our parents we were to do it on Saturday. Again, I was worried. More 'telling' Mum what had to happen, and I was not allowed out on Saturdays anyway. But I thought what fun it would be if she let me do this.

I ran all the way home as before and told Mum, 'The policeman said . . .' She looked very doubtful and told me she would speak to Dad. Luckily, he was quite enthusiastic, saying that it was a useful thing for me to do for the war effort.

I had been paired with a cheery girl, and she came to the school on Saturday morning with a rickety old pram and we set off. It was great to be allowed to go round knocking on people's doors— a thing normally frowned on—and trundling the old pram about the village. After the first surprised look, people were delighted to get rid of a lot of their old junk, and we soon had a pram full of clanking forks, trowels, buckets (buckets were all made of metal), saucepans, frying pans, old knives, tin paint pots, a few tin toys and a tin bath—this had to be balanced precariously on top of the pram. Everything was old or broken and, for the most part, rusty.

On the way back to the school with our load, a wheel came off the pram. It tipped over, and everything fell out with a fearful clatter and my partner had to chase the wheel down the high street. At first, we laughed about it but then wondered how we were going to get all this stuff to the school.

Mr. Williams came out of his shop, having heard the noise. 'Youm in a mess, girls. After the shop shuts, I'll mend the pram for you.'

This was very kind, but the shop didn't close until six p.m. We had to be back at the school by four p.m. We piled all that we could into the tin bath and tried to lift it to the school . . . but it was far too heavy! Out came half the goods, which we stacked in the broken pram, and, leaving it on the pavement by the shop, we made for school with the half-full old bath between us. The policeman was there with a small lorry. He took the scrap, and when he heard our tale of woe, he told us to jump into the cab and show him where we had left the rest. This was great fun. We were riding high up in the lorry, grinning at all the others who were tramping towards the school by now.

Mr. Williams mended the pram and kept it for us for the next Saturday. We started to 'do' the houses that we had had to leave in 'our' area, but soon there were shouts from the ones we had visited last week. Most people had been inspired to clear out sheds and cupboards, gardens and garages, and had piles of metal objects for us. We thought they were very generous, but when I told Dad he wagged his head.

'They will be only too glad to get rid of old stuff that has been piling up for years,' he said. 'The dustmen won't take that sort of thing, so you kids are a godsend.'

Of course, there were no recycling centres or 'dumps' as there are now, and disposing of large objects was a real problem.

The policeman was pleased with us all and even extended the Scrap Iron Drive for two more Saturdays. It was good fun: Mum even seemed interested in what I was doing, so I was allowed to tell Grandma and Granddad S. all about it at the tea table. Granddad was shocked that the government was having to 'beg', as he put it, but Dad said that anything to help get rid of Hitler was not begging.

A week or two later, some men went around the village cutting off people's iron garden railings. I don't think the owner's permission was asked: the railings were just 'commandeered' by the authorities, we were told. There are many gardens in the country which still bear the evidence: stubby bits of metal can be seen protruding from the garden walls where there were once quite intricately patterned railings.

The Country Nurse Remembers

Another war effort the children were involved in was the *concert*. Any child who could recite a poem, sing a song, play the piano or do anything entertaining was told that there would be rehearsals the following day.

A friend Sheila and I were to sing a duet of 'The White Cliffs of Dover', while two sisters were singing and playing the piano at the same time. We were impressed by this. I was to play the only piano piece that I knew—I had only been going to the piano teacher for a few weeks. She lived in a dark, cold house near the school, and I went there on Friday afternoons after lessons. I was frightened of her. She was very impatient, which made me jittery. Perhaps I was a slow learner—and I probably had little real talent.

The whole class was going to open *and close* the concert with the national anthem (Governess was very patriotic) and sing some wartime songs and a few hymns. David—of pilot's thumb fame—was eager to juggle three tennis balls but had lost one. We were told to hunt about at home to try to find one for him, as this was an unusual act. Another boy showed Governess how he could walk on his hands—legs waving uncertainly in the air—but she felt that he might kick somebody in the audience, so he settled for rolling over and over in circles. Lots of children opted to recite a poem, and the little ones from the other class were going to do a dance. We were all excited and kept coming up with more and more bizarre ideas for the parents' entertainment.

At last, Governess had worked out the order of appearances, with the little ones performing near the beginning so that they could go home to bed. We spent all the afternoon rehearsing and then were instructed to go home and tell our parents to come to this great concert. Oh dear! More *telling*.

This time I was not so clever.

'There's a concert for the parents next Tuesday at six p.m.,' I said to Mum.

She was at the cooker. 'Oh! Well, I don't think your dad and I will be going to that. Just get your shoes cleaned and lay the table.'

I was disappointed to think that they would not hear Sheila and me sing or see the other acts.

'Sheila and I are going to sing at the concert.'

'What concert?'

'The concert next Tuesday for the parents.'

'You are supposed to sing?'

'Yes. Lots of us are doing things.'

She frowned. 'Oh, I don't think we can let you do that. I'm sure Dad would not like you doing that.'

I was nearly sick. Not only was I bitterly disappointed that I would not be part of this great event, but I couldn't imagine how I was going to tell Governess and, worse still, the other children. I did my chores, puzzling and worrying. Why was Dad likely to object, and why did they not even want to come? I hid my tears. I wondered why I did not let Mum see how upset I was. Would it have made any difference?

Later, Mum and Dad sat me in front of them and questioned me. What was this concert all about? I told them it was part of the war effort and would cost them sixpence each to get in. Why had I not *asked* if I might do this singing and so on rather than just saying that I was *going* to do it? I said that we were all told what we were to do: Governess said so.

'Very high-handed,' said Mum. 'And what makes you think you can sing?'

I didn't know what to say to this. Mum obviously did not think that I could sing, so how could I reply without contradicting? I did what I always resorted to in such difficulties: I said, 'I don't know.'

'Huh,' said Mum. 'Well, you'd make a fool of yourself, and poor Sheila.'

Surprisingly, Dad spoke up. 'Oh, I don't know. None of the kids are likely to be much better. I suppose we'd better let her do it. And I think we should go, just to support the war effort.'

I began to hope.

'Waste of time, I reckon,' Mum muttered.

Gradually, I gathered that not only could I take part, but they would also come to the concert. I was so glad that I would not have to tell everyone that I couldn't do it. Though now I was worried in case I *was* going to make a fool of myself, as Mum had said. For the first time in my life, I experienced stage fright, although I did not know what to call the butterflies that seemed to have taken up residence in my tummy. Before, it had just been fun and exciting.

Later in his life, Dad did a lot of singing, solo and choral, and was very confident. I have never been able to understand why there was a problem about me appearing on stage and why he, as well as Mum, seemed ashamed of the idea.

We rehearsed several times, and then Tuesday arrived. The screen wall had been pushed back by a grumbling boiler man, and two double desks had been placed together to make a sort of tiny stage for the children who were to sing solos or duets. There was a chair beside the desk for us to climb up.

The parents all sat in rows on small school chairs. The big, tall dads looked funny—they didn't seem to know what to do with their long legs.

Governess said a few words and then played the piano for everyone, parents included, to sing the national anthem. The little ones did their dance, most of them forgetting what they were supposed to do, but the parents clapped, and many of these tiny ones were taken home to bed. The class sang various songs, and then it was Sheila and me. We climbed onto the desk, Governess played the introduction and we sang 'The White Cliffs of Dover'. We didn't go wrong, and we were clapped enthusiastically. I thought that I hadn't made a fool of myself after all. My piano playing was much less accomplished, but I still got through my one and only tune.

The boys did their tricks and marched up and down in step to some marching music that Governess played. There were various recitations, and then the class sang a hymn. Governess stood up and thanked the parents for coming and for their money towards the war effort—I don't remember what it was supposed to pay for—and then everyone stood for the national anthem once again.

Lots of parents stood about for a bit, chatting while the children started to put the chairs back into place. The grumpy boiler man appeared and pulled the screen across and shuffled the desks about, and it was all over.

On the way home, I heard Dad say that he was surprised how clear my voice was. Mum didn't say that I had made a fool of myself, and so I wondered if, perhaps, I *could* sing after all.

The last of our war efforts was a gym display. We did not do gym as we know it now, we just did exercises: running on the spot and a lot of jumping in the playground, with Governess standing in the shelter of the doorway, in her suit and court shoes, shouting the orders and clapping her hands for us to keep time. This happened about three times a week. Sometimes we played with a ball to 'improve our reactions', said Governess, and sometimes there were team games. There was no room for races or anything elaborate, so the gym display was not very exciting, but it posed more problems at home.

The school had a number of 'daps' (light, thin canvas shoes) of different sizes, and when we did gym we just chose a pair in the right size and put them back into the shoebox afterwards. Luckily these boxes were in the cloakrooms, so the boys' shoes were separate from ours. The girls were sure that the boys' shoes would smell, as we were convinced that all boys had smelly feet. None of this seems very hygienic these days, but I think it was done this way because some families might not have been able to afford gym shoes for their fast-growing children. When clothes rationing came, it was probably impossible to spare precious coupons for such shoes anyway.

'We are giving a gym display,' I told Mum.

'Have we got to come to that?'

'No, it's for the vicar and a lot of important men.'

'When? I hope it's in school time.'

'Yes—on Friday.'

Mum thought for a while. 'I suppose you'd better wear your school summer sandals for that.'

'No, we are wearing blue shoes.'

'What blue shoes? It's no good you thinking you are going to get new shoes just for a gym display. We don't have coupons to spare for that sort of nonsense. Blue shoes indeed!' Mum paused for breath.

'School shoes,' I said quickly, before she could start to grumble again.

'What?'

So I explained about the school shoes that we all shared.

'And you have been wearing these shoes for gym all this time and you didn't tell me!'

I didn't know what to say. It had just never come up. Dad and Mum rarely asked anything about what we did at school.

'Everybody has to wear them for gym . . . ' I said tentatively. Then I had a sudden inspiration. 'Governess says.'

'Hmm. I still think I should have been told.'

I was trying to smooth things over without knowing why Mum was cross.

'We wear our own socks,' I said. I didn't know if this was a good thing or if it would make her even more cross. 'And the shoes are washed at the end of term.' I was not even sure if this was true or not. They looked cleaner at the beginning of term than at the end, but I think I was becoming devious and scarcely truthful. I was afraid that once more there would be problems about me doing the display.

Even now, I do not know why she was so angry. We were not a super-fussy family, and even two girls from a really posh family in the village used the shoes.

Our timid vicar seemed nervous but smiled at the display, which he watched with about eight important-looking men in suits and trilby hats. We were told that they were the school governors. I didn't know we had any; as far as I was concerned we just had Governess.

Good Intentions

It seemed that Mum had never got on very well with her mother, Grandma S. They were very different. Mum prided herself on being down to earth, whereas Grandma said Mum was living in another era.

Grandma had been brought up in a big, fairly wealthy family on the Isle of Wight. I don't think the family liked her marrying Granddad, who was a Royal Marine, but not a very high-ranking one. Grandma seemed to cling to old-fashioned ways and did not realise that money was short and rationing was a problem. She wanted fancy food and liked posh clothes and expensive perfumes.

She did see that some of the things Mum expected of me were unreasonable, however. I heard her say this to Mum one day, but I knew it would do more harm than good. She went on to say that it was ridiculous for a child to have to knock on doors and wait to be told to come in in her own home. Mum pursed her lips and told me to go and play. Then there was a lot of shouting, which I could hear from the garden.

Later, when I was in the other room, I heard Granddad, who hardly even spoke to me, say that I should not be banished to the other room or sent off to bed at such a 'ridiculously early hour'.

I know they were trying to help me, but I also knew that Mum would resent their interference—just as she had when Grandpa had tried to help me.

Mum was very angry and told Dad what they had said in such a way that he thought it was just interference, too. He always thought that Mum knew best about everything to do with my upbringing and didn't seem to notice that she was always telling me off, never praising me, sending me away to the other room or the garden or to bed, or making me spend Saturdays doing housework. He just did not notice that I hardly spoke when Mum was around except to say 'yes' or 'thank you' and so on. So he sided with Mum against Grandma and Granddad, saying that they were in 'his house' and they should not interfere.

Mum was very cross with everyone except Dad.

'You realise that all this is your fault, don't you?' she said to me.

As always, I had to say, 'Yes Mum. I'm sorry, Mum.' But I couldn't see how it could be my fault.

Dad looked at her a bit oddly but said nothing.

How I wished that Harry was still living with us! But he would have been in Dad's house too, of course, so he might have been told he was just interfering, as well.

I must have been very stupid because only a few days after this I asked if I could write to Auntie Jinny. Why did I not wait a week or two?

'Why?' asked Mum.

'I'd just like to,' I replied.

'What are you going to say to her?'

'Um . . . just about the war effort at school and things.'

'Well, all right, but I want to see what you've written before you put it in the envelope.'

The Country Nurse Remembers

There was a lot of huffing while Mum found a writing pad, gave me one sheet and an envelope. I turned to go in the other room.

'You had better sit at the table to write this letter,' instructed Mum.

With Mum watching me, it took me a long time to think what to write, and I made it a very short letter. It was a bit messy because the pencil broke and we could not find the pencil sharpener. Dad came in about then and sharpened the pencil with a knife, and I was able to write the ending, which had to be very formal: 'Your loving great-niece, Julia.' Only I couldn't spell 'niece' and had to rub it out when Mum pointed out my mistake and that made another splodge.

'Well, what a mess!' said Mum, looking at the letter. 'I don't think we can send that.' And she took the envelope away and screwed up the letter.

I cried that night. I had so wanted to feel in contact with Auntie Jinny. I knew that she wrote sometimes, but the mail was addressed to Dad and Mum, and I was not told what the letter said. She would not have written just to me—that was not the way in those days; a letter had to be to the parents with, perhaps, a message or 'love' to a child. But while I expect Auntie Jinny did send love, I was never told.

I was such a wimp that I did not try to write again—it caused too much of a fuss.

The Great Escape—That Wasn't

I don't think it could have been because of the 'interference row', but soon Grandma went off to stay with her friend in the house next door to their own, and shortly afterwards Granddad followed. It seemed that they were going to have a couple of rooms and either rent or lodge (I was not sure what the difference was) in that house instead of at Meadow View. Grandma had never liked the fact that we were in the country and rather isolated compared with their home in Bath. Now she would be back on familiar ground.

There was another reason for the move, too. Their house, although not officially fit for habitation, was being lived in *un*officially by a lady and her children who were squatting. Dad explained that many people whose houses had been completely demolished and were homeless had found damaged homes that had been abandoned but were just about safe and had moved in. Granddad had to see solicitors and the authorities, because he had heard that once someone occupied a house in this way it was difficult to make them move out, although they were not paying rent or anything. It was evidently very worrying, and Granddad said he would rather be nearby to keep an eye on the situation.

The Country Nurse Remembers

So apart from Granddad's piano, which would not fit in their rooms and so stayed at Meadow View, the house was back to normal: rather empty and very quiet. I had liked having more people around, and the disruption of my rigid routine had given me a little more freedom and alleviated my loneliness—or perhaps my *aloneness*.

The war effort weeks had done much to make things more interesting too, and I had enjoyed being out and about with other children.

In contrast, Mum seemed to like things being back to normal and redoubled her efforts to ensure that I did everything exactly as she wanted and as fast as possible. I was also back to bed early, whether in the shelter or in my room, and once more was not allowed to get up in the holidays until Mum called, which was often so late in the morning.

Looking back now, I find it difficult to imagine how I amused myself in bed from six in the evening until about ten the following morning, with no books or drawing equipment, dolls or teddies, and no drink of water. The window overlooked the garden, but once in bed I had to lie still and was not allowed to sit up to look outside. There were no pictures on the walls; in fact, the only way that anyone would know that it was my room as opposed to anyone else's was that my hairbrush was on the dressing table. Otherwise the room could have been empty—unoccupied.

Even the bed had to be made so carefully that it did not look as though anyone had slept in it. There were no duvets; we had sheets and blankets with an eiderdown for cold nights. I almost preferred the shelter because it was darker, and so I think I went to sleep more quickly, and occasionally, in the morning, Tig might wander in from the garden.

Perhaps it was the contrast between the bustle of the full house (in a way, I had mattered more then and felt properly useful) and the return of the old routine that made me particularly aware of a kind of dreariness, a hopelessness. Nothing was ever going to change.

How I wished I were still a five-year-old with a 'real' Mummy. If only the last five years had not happened at all and I was that little girl who had been loved. I don't know that I thought it all out exactly like this, but this was the gist of my ramblings. I remembered that Mum had said that no one would want me when I grew up, and I supposed that was just the way it was going to be. It did not occur to me that she might be wrong.

I began to wish that I knew how children ran away. You heard stories at school about such children, and they always ended up somewhere wonderful or came home to loving arms.

Suddenly, for no reason, I remembered the stories that Mummy used to tell me. I had completely forgotten about them. It made me realise that no one had ever read to me since her death.

I was now able to read for myself and enjoyed the books at school, but the only books I had at home were girls' annuals, which seemed to be about the sort of girls who were pretty and clever, lived in big houses and had wonderful toys. I had never met anyone remotely like these girls. I also had Rupert annuals, which I loved—probably because they were about animals, imaginary animals. They are the only fantasy type of book that I have ever liked; tales about fairies were silly, I thought, and yet I did not think Rupert so. Not very logical . . . Eventually I began to be given Enid Blyton books and much, much later Arthur Ransome books. These seemed real, as they were about children who had adventures. How I envied them!

Since my grandparents and Harry had left, my life had become dreary again, and I was suffocated by all Mum's restrictions. I longed for company, but I had to play by myself in the other room.

In there were two big cupboards built either side of the chimney breast. The left-hand one was divided so that the top part had crockery and such things in it and the bottom part was my toy cupboard. It was deep and came up to the height of the mantlepiece. It had a shelf, and the floor was like another shelf. With the doors wide open, I played with dolls, dressing and undressing them, giving them a 'life', pretending that the shelf was their home, while I sat on a small stool in front of the cupboard. If I wanted to draw or read my annuals, I put all the doll things on the floor under the shelf and spread my books, pencils and drawing paper out on top, but it was often rather dark in the corner and there was not enough light to see properly. I once asked if I might sit on the settee and do my drawing on my lap but was told that I would only spread all my things about and that would make the place untidy. I was so . . . what was I? Fed up? Low? Depressed? I didn't know. And I didn't know these words, either—I was just the way I was.

One of the things that happened about then was that I only just saved all my dolls from being given away. I knew I should give toys to poor children who had been bombed out and had none, but I only just got home in time to save Margaret from the pile that Mum had collected while I was at school. *All* my dolls were in a heap on the settee when I got back.

'We are going to give them to Barnardo's. They are appealing for toys.'

I was aghast! 'Please, please may I keep Margaret? And . . . and Baby?'

I held my breath, as Mum thought for a moment. 'Well, I suppose you could. And that other baby doll is not worth sending.'

Tiggy had chewed the doll in question when he was a puppy, but I was glad to add her to the other two.

I was so relieved. 'All the rest can go,' I said, 'and the farm animals and the annuals.' I rushed to give all sorts away. I was sorry for these children and wanted to give them things, but I just loved these three dolls—they were a part of the time before my mother died. I was sure that Mum would have given them all away had I not returned from school just in time.

Then there was something else. Something that hurt more than anything else because it was not Mum being mean; it was *Dad*.

On my way into the house after school one day soon after the doll episode, I glanced into the greenhouse. My doll's house was missing! It was small—only about a foot across—but Mum had never allowed it in the house: it stood against the back wall of the house in the lean-to greenhouse, so I only played with it if the weather was not too cold or too hot. But I loved to wallpaper the tiny rooms, build stairs from matchboxes, make little bed covers and bring the miniature dolls to life.

'Mum, where has my doll's house gone?'

Mum was cooking. She did not usually even look round when I came in, but today she turned round and looked directly at me. She took a big breath.

'I'm afraid your dad has sold it. I didn't know or I would have stopped him.'

I was stunned. 'Why, Mum?'

'Dad's selling the car. A man came to see it and said he would buy it if Dad included the doll's house. By the time I knew, it was too late. I know you still play with it.'

I cried then. I felt bereft. I had loved that doll's house. How could Dad do this to me? One good thing was that Mum was on my side for once, but she was cross with Dad and that was *not* good.

She sighed and said, 'I'm sorry.' Here was Mum saying 'sorry' to me! For Dad, I supposed. I thought Dad would have said 'sorry' too, but he said nothing until the next day.

'I didn't think you played with that doll's house,' he said. 'It's always in the greenhouse.'

The Country Nurse Remembers

At first I didn't understand. It *lived* in the greenhouse. It was never anywhere else.

'I play with it there,' I said.

'I didn't know that. Why?'

'That's where it lives.'

Dad had never noticed that the doll's house never came into the house . . . that I played with it in the greenhouse. I didn't know what to think or feel. I was so unhappy that he had done this to me: that mattered more than the loss of the doll's house itself.

I brooded for the rest of the week. I wanted things to be different, but how could they be? I didn't know. And what was the alternative? Some children ran away. How did they do that? I had no idea. I spent time dreaming and planning . . . planning what exactly I could not have said, but when I set off for Sunday school that week I stopped before reaching the gates to the church and turned off into the fields. I was crying, frightened about what I was doing, but a little bit excited, too. I walked to the first gate and into the next field. There were cows there. I liked cows, and these were quietly chewing their cuds and watching me with their big, soft eyes. I went near them and talked to them. One of them mooed back, and I sat down on the grass and looked at them all. Then I looked at the fields, stretching away into the distance. I thought of the trouble I'd be in if I ran away and was brought back—and I knew I'd be brought back because I had no idea how to go about this business of running away. I had nowhere to go, no one near enough to go to and, in any case, they would just send me home.

I got up and turned back. I was a failure: I knew that. It had been a silly idea, anyway. Had I only been pretending? I wondered. I would never have had the courage to go through with such a plan. Plan? There was no plan.

I skulked near the church until I saw the children come out. I waited until they had dispersed and then ran home. Until now, no one has ever known of my pathetic attempt at running away.

Prisoners of War

I knew that Dad had been having great difficulties at the Works. He only had three of the original twelve men to do all the work, and the bombing in Bath and its surrounds meant extra hours overseeing new pipework or repairs, involving many trips into the city. He employed a tiny old man who had retired from the Works several years earlier but was glad to 'get out missus's road'. Dad gave him the easier jobs and found him useful, but the maintenance of roads, trees, hedges and verges could not be fitted in, and the bomb blasts had shattered a lot of windows, which needed to be repaired.

The 'powers that be', Dad said, would have to find him some more men from somewhere. And, apparently, they did.

One morning—it must have been holiday time—an old army lorry trundled past the house on the way to the Works.

'What the . . . ?' Dad was into his jacket and on with his hat and after it in no time.

A while later, he came back to say that the corporation had sent him some German prisoners of war to do some of the heavy work.

Mum was nervous. 'Are they all right? Not dangerous?'

Dad said that a soldier with a gun was in charge of them but seemed to think that they would not be a problem.

All Mum could say was 'Hmm.'

'What do they look like, Dad?' I asked.

'Just like anyone else,' he replied. 'Did you think they might have two heads or something?'

He was only joking, but I didn't like it when Mum or Dad made fun of me. Perhaps it was because I was not usually given the chance to explain what I had meant—as now. I had wondered if they were huge or ugly, if they had bandages on, if they had horrible tempers or if they smiled. I couldn't think that they *would* smile—they were prisoners, after all, weren't they?

The next day Dad appeared at the back door with one of the prisoners.

'It's all right,' he said, and he told us the man's name, though I don't remember what it was. The man was light-haired and not very tall. He looked young for a soldier—more like a senior schoolboy. He had two pairs of slippers in his hand. They were made from several different colours of string. He offered the small pair to me. I shrank back, thinking that I would not be allowed to take them. But he jabbered something and smiled, and then he kind of bowed to Mum and gave her both pairs. He bowed again and went out of the door. The soldier, 'one of our Tommies', was waiting for him with his rifle slung over his shoulder on a strap. The rest of the prisoners were in the back of the truck.

They had all been allocated jobs the day before and shown what needed doing, and now they were to be set to work again. Dad said they were good workers, but he didn't seem very happy. Evidently people in the village did not like having the prisoners nearby and blamed Dad, saying that he was being unpatriotic. Dad was furious and had what he called a 'set-to' with a few of the village men who did not seem to realise that the scheme was making good use of prison labour.

'You'd think they would be glad to know that these POWs were doing something to earn their keep rather than sitting on their bottoms at our expense!' Dad raged on.

The prisoners made the slippers and other things and sold them for pennies to buy cigarettes. I was surprised at first that Dad was willing to give them money, but I suppose we needed slippers, and these would not be on coupons. They were surprisingly comfortable and lasted a long time.

We rarely, if ever, heard the word 'Nazi'—to us children the Germans were known as 'Huns', 'Crouts' or 'the Axis' (with the other countries fighting against us), 'Hitler's lot' or just plain 'the enemy'. Now, when the Second World War is mentioned, we talk about Nazis, or Nazi Germany, but during the war years local people did not make any distinction between the German people and the Nazis. There was really no distinction to *be* made, as the Nazis had such a stranglehold on the German nation that decent Germans had no voice at all. It was only after the war, when we watched films or documentaries or read wartime history, that we understood this.

The prisoners' work enabled Dad to catch up on all the jobs that had been left unattended, but his relationship with the village was strained. I was not aware of this personally, but Mum and Dad worried about it. I don't remember how long the Germans stayed, but I think it was only a few weeks, and, apart from the man with the slippers, I only caught glimpses of them as they were driven past.

Mum was uneasy and said that she didn't want them anywhere near the house. Dad tried to understand them (they spoke a little English) to see why they were fighting for a man like Hitler. He said that some of them didn't seem to know why they were fighting at all but that one had started to shout 'Heil Hitler'. The Tommy raised his gun and pointed it at the man and told Dad not to talk to any of the prisoners at all in future in case there was trouble. Dad was relieved when they went but wondered how he would manage without them.

A Wartime Birthday

Obviously, I must have had birthdays during the war, but, apart from one—perhaps my tenth—I do not remember them. I think most parents tried to make children's birthdays special, but it was not easy. Birthday cakes, if made at all, would have to be eggless and almost sugarless; icing was just not possible, as the sugar ration was meagre, and candles were a thing of the past. Jelly was still available, and, as long as you had milk, you could make custard. Pastry took rather too much fat, so fancy tarts were out of the question for parties—mine, anyway (pastry was for apple tarts and other filling puddings). About the only sandwich fillings were fish paste or spam. This strange meat was fairly readily available, and all the youngsters liked it. Granddad S. said it 'was not fit to eat, as you didn't know what was in it'. I think there were many foods on the market during and after the war, including horse meat and whale meat, that were labelled as something else.

I was as keen as any other child to have a party until I really thought about it. All the others had some sort of 'tea', so I wanted to be seen to have one, too. But I was always on edge in case one of my four or five school friends said something to get me into trouble.

I always felt more freedom in school and often broke some of Mum's rules about putting on my hat and coat for playtime or keeping the elasticated legs of my knickers down almost to the hem of my skirt. I pulled them up out of sight as soon as I was anywhere near school. The teasing would have been too awful! Or perhaps I played with some child whose parents Mum and Dad didn't like. There were all sorts of things that my friends might have talked about within Mum's hearing, and I wonder now that I was so keen to have a 'tea'. I suppose it was worth the risk just to be like everyone else.

When we went to each other's houses for a tea (or a proper party sometimes), we took our slippers. This was always the done thing: a small present and your slippers. At the end, the host child would say, 'Thank you for coming and don't forget your slippers.'

'Thank you for having me and I've got my slippers,' we would reply. It was always the same: rather stilted but polite. Quite different from the way we communicated in the playground!

I believe everyone takes home 'party bags' these days, but there was no such thing then. We did not decorate the house for the event either, but it is possible that some folk had a few balloons, though *they* were almost unobtainable once the war came. Any rubber that 'got through' (on the ships) was needed for army lorry tyres, we were told.

We played very ordinary games—hunt the slipper, hide-and-seek, statues (if someone could play the piano) and pin the tail on the donkey. Donkeys were of the oddest shapes, as the child concerned drew and painted it herself. Pass the parcel was nearly all wrapping, with a tiny present, perhaps an apple, inside. In our house, we had to have 'hunt the thimble' because our games were confined to the 'other room', so something as large as a slipper would soon have been found. Hide-and-seek was only possible in good weather, but my birthday was in the winter.

The Country Nurse Remembers

Mum kept stern watch over the tea table but cleared up and washed up afterwards, leaving us to play in the other room.

'You are so different when your mother is around,' a friend said.

'No, I'm not,' I answered, in my usual prickly way.

I so wanted to be like everyone else that I deluded myself. The girl concerned was probably only being friendly or was genuinely puzzled.

When the party was over, the children would have trudged off along the dark lane to their homes in the village. The country was a much safer place for children then than it is now, but Dad worried about the river if there had been a lot of rain, as there *had* been on this birthday: the lane was prone to flood very quickly. So he piled all the children into the car (no seat belts in those days) and drove them up the hill and into the village, where they all got out and dispersed. I would have liked to have gone too, but I had to clear up.

There were a number of fish-paste sandwiches left over, as they were not a favourite, so I had to eat them for breakfast the next morning. I did not tell my friends that. My breakfast was usually a jam sandwich, but now and again we had porridge, which I loved. Dad kept bees, and so we had honey on the porridge instead of sugar. It was very tasty.

Words, Words, Words

The language of war, like war itself, somehow infiltrated our consciousness, and a whole new vocabulary opened up to us. It was all everyone talked about—well, the grown-ups certainly—so to gain any understanding we had to guess at what words meant and hope for the best.

The 'black market' was not a market at all, it seemed, black or otherwise, but just a name given to goods that people sold without coupons. Were the goods black, or were the people selling them black? Were the people black, hence the name? I had only seen one black person thus far in my life. He had appeared in the village one day, as the school was coming out.

Then we heard of a country called 'Russia'. 'Communists' lived there and were fighting the Germans because Hitler had been silly enough to start a second front—whatever that was. Communists wore ragged clothes and didn't have enough guns, but the cold winter helped them. This was a mystery.

Dad said that Tom, his friend the farmer, had had one of his lorries commandeered by the army. Tom was upset but had said, 'If they want it, they'd better have it.' What was that all about?

There was a great song, 'We're Going to Hang Out the Washing on the Siegfried Line'. I knew that it was *not* a washing line, but I was almost an adult before I learned that it was a German defence line, built in the First World War and reinstated in the Second World War. The song implied that it would not hold out against the Allies for long, so it made people feel cheerful.

We heard that spies 'infiltrated' the enemy, that the Germans were 'anti-Semitic'—was this a disease? And the 'French Resistance' helped airmen who had been shot down. I don't think I understood that France had been conquered by Germany and went on 'resisting'. People said that France had 'capitulated'; they were very scathing about this. I couldn't understand it at all—had they been conquered or had they capitulated? And what was the difference?

Some people were making a lot of money, making guns and things, and this was 'profiteering'. It was evidently not right.

Although I still listened to the six o'clock news on Fridays, I only understood about the fighting—and that not very well. I just knew that we lost some battles and won some, that Montgomery was a great soldier, that lots of soldiers were killed and that Mr. Churchill was directing the war: 'We shall fight on the beaches. We shall fight in the fields and in the streets. We shall fight in the hills. We shall never surrender.' People loved Mr. Churchill and were quite sure that he would win the war for us. The vicar was quite cross at one of the Thursday services when one of the boys said that Mr. Churchill was so clever.

'Remember,' he said, 'that God is directing Mr. Churchill. Without God's help, we will not win the war.'

None of us had the slightest doubt that God was on our side, so how could we lose? So why was everyone so worried? It was all very confusing.

Sometimes, I would ask Dad what something meant and he'd try to explain, but he was always so tired that Mum said to let him be. So I lived in a sort of bubble of ignorance, and my own small life just plodded along.

I never did find out what a 'quisling' was. I formed the impression that it was a kind of eel, for some reason. It did not occur to me that it was the name of a person, and in any case the word entered the language very quickly to mean a traitor.

I think many children had very odd ideas about the rights and wrongs of the war: the principles, honour, intrigue. And Hitler himself, and Mussolini in Italy. Some of my friends were better informed by their parents, but now that the heavy bombing had almost stopped (there were still raids on Bristol but not so often), the war did not seem to affect us children so much. We were used to rationing and being told not to show a light and to dig for victory and 'do our bit' for the war effort and not to talk to strangers in case they were German spies. We accepted the darkness everywhere, now that there were no streetlights. Our lane had never had them anyway, but the village had been lit. There were no road or town names and no signposts; they had all been removed at the beginning of the war to confuse the Germans, had they invaded. Dad knew the local area and nearby towns and roads well, and, in any case, we did not go far from home during the war.

A New Teacher

Life went on as usual—until one day we went to school and Governess was not there. She had apparently retired.

No one had told us or our parents that this was imminent. There was no big send-off, Governess did not get a retirement gift and there was nothing in the papers about her long service to education. It was all a bit sudden. Maybe she wanted it this way, or perhaps it was just one more result of the war, meaning that people were busy trying to keep their families fed and clothed, and so poor Governess just disappeared. I think her husband retired at the same time, and the village hardly ever saw them from then on.

Miss Martin, the new teacher, stood at the front of our class on the first morning of the term. She was much younger than Governess; probably in her mid-twenties. She had hair done in a modern style, whereas Governess had had a bun. Miss Martin's clothes were more up to date, and she wore lipstick. Whilst widely used, lipstick, on a teacher, was a surprise to us, as Governess had not worn make-up at all.

'Good morning children,' Miss Martin said.

We answered as we always had: 'Good morning, Governess.'

She looked rather shocked. 'Oh no,' she said. 'I do not wish to be called "Governess". You will call me Miss Martin.'

We said, 'Yes, Miss Martin.'

Miss Martin's way of teaching us was very different from Governess's rather stiff, precise way. She encouraged us to discuss things to do with the war. Perhaps Mr. Churchill's latest speech, or some battle, or why a certain ship had been sunk. We were used to the school curriculum of reading, writing and arithmetic, with some history and nature study and instruction in good manners. The girls learnt to knit while the boys did things with cardboard and glue (when it was available), and we did gym. But that was all. Discussion was new. The boys loved talking about the war, and Miss Martin seemed to listen to them and then either agree or disagree. The girls were more inclined to talk about the way that the war was affecting their homes, and Miss Martin was equally interested, offering some opinions herself. She then told us where she had been teaching before, where she was living now, a bit about her parents and her brother. It was all very chatty and rather confusing for us after Governess's rigid discipline.

Mum and Dad looked sceptical when I told them about it all. They seemed to think that all this 'chat' was a waste of learning time. I suppose 'modern' methods of teaching were being introduced, and many parents were worried that discipline and respect for elders was being undermined. I didn't know what all that meant, but I think Miss Martin had a struggle to convince them that encouraging us to think for ourselves *was* part of teaching. Mum certainly would not have approved, as she did not like me to think for myself. She had always said that she would tell me what to think.

After a few weeks, some parents were disturbed by a rumour that Miss Martin had been seen out walking in the evening with a young man. They seemed to find this worrying in itself, and then someone noticed that the young man was not in uniform. Rumours buzzed about. Was he a conchie? And if so, should Miss Martin, who might have 'radical ideas'—whatever those were—be teaching impressionable young children?

These whisperings eventually reached Miss Martin's ears, and she took the unusual step of refuting them head on. One day, she stood in front of the top class and told us to inform our parents that the young man, with whom she had been walking, was her brother, who was still at university but would be joining up when he left next year, if the war was not over by then. We were very impressed, partly because she had told us such personal things and because she had a brother at university. Most of us did not know anyone who was at university and, at this early stage in our education, could not imagine that any of us would ever get to those dizzying heights of cleverness.

The school continued to suffer shortages. There was often no paper on which to write or draw, and we had no pencil sharpeners. If we had a broken pencil or crayon, we had to take it home and get it sharpened, perhaps with a kitchen knife or a penknife. Before my time, children had written on slates with chalk, so now the slates were unearthed, some chalk found and we all had to do spellings and sums on them instead. It was very messy, made worse by 'rubbings out' with a well-licked finger.

The heating was often not working because there was no coal for the furnace, so we were told to keep our coats and gloves on. Writing on slate with chalk in woolly gloves was not easy, but Miss Martin insisted that by not complaining we were helping the war effort. I wondered how the war people, like Mr. Churchill, would manage. David said that they would have lots of paper and proper fountain pens and they would be sitting in great big warm rooms. However, we preferred to think of Mr. Churchill in woolly gloves, with chalk on his cigar.

Mice Galore

I had now had mice for many months, perhaps a year, and during that time there had been a population explosion among them.

After the arrival of Winnie and Bobbie's family, Dad said that we would have to separate the boys from the girls as soon as they were old enough. But no one knew how old they had to be before they could be taken from their mother, or how to tell boys from girls. Mice are very small, and even though Mum and Dad upended the little things and stared hard at their 'underneath bits', they could not see any difference. I suppose these days one would take them to a vet, who would know straight away, but people did not use vets as often as they do now, and certainly not for such a thing as this. Neither did we know how old they had to be before they started families of their own. Well, we were soon to find out.

Dad had only just started to make another mouse box when we found that Winnie and Bobbie had had another family. The first family had been housed in a cardboard box whilst waiting for their new home, but there must have been boys and girls together because we found *two* new families in there, as well. Dad brought Mr. Burn in to try to 'sex' them. This was probably the first time that I had heard this word, but, because of the context, I more or less knew its meaning, and I was very embarrassed to think that

The Country Nurse Remembers

Mr. Burn was involved. Between him, Dad and Mum, the boys were identified and removed to a different box, and Dad started to make about six more homes for all the mice. He was quite happy doing this, but it must have been a nuisance, as he was so busy at the Works. Mum found bits of old cloth for bedding, and all the mouse houses were put on a wide shelf in the greenhouse. The windows had been partially blown out by the blast of bombs, so Dad said they would have plenty of fresh air.

We kept lots of logs for the fire on the floor under the shelf. One day, I went to feed all these mice, clean them out and give them fresh water, and I found that my original and favourite two, Winnie and Bobbie, had escaped. I called Mum, who came to help me look for them. We realised that they must be in among all these logs. When Dad came home, he said that the only way to get them to come out was to get some bits of meat or something that smelled good and put it in their cage, which should be put on the floor with the door open so that the mouse would smell the food, go to eat it and, when it entered the cage, we could quickly shut the door.

So we took turns at watching for the returning escapees. I had my teatime sandwiches watching. It got dark, so I got a torch and went on watching. At last there was a shuffling, and a little white figure ran into the cage and began to eat the meat. I crept forward and shut the cage door. Winnie was safe!

Now we had to get Bobbie.

Some more meat was put in a big glass jar, which was placed on its side, and we waited for him to appear. Nothing happened.

It was long past my bedtime, so Mum said they would go on watching for him and I should go to bed. I had school the next day. Mum and Dad seemed worried about Bobbie in case he had gone altogether, so I knew they would go on watching for 'that scallywag', as Dad called him.

The next morning, both the mice were together in their cage. Dad had gone to work, but Mum told me that they had watched for a long time, and, though Bobbie had peeped out of the logs, he had not been interested in the meat. So Dad had had the idea of putting the flashlight behind Winnie, in her cage, so that Bobbie could see her. It worked, and Bobbie soon crept out from the logs and ran to the cage to be with Winnie. Mum quickly grabbed him, opened the cage, popped him in, shut the door, gave them some food and the hunt was over. I was very happy to know that the mice were safe, and I had a sort of warm feeling because Dad and Mum had been so glad to help me.

However, none of us had realised that the boy mice would fight, so *they* had to be parted. More boxes! Some mistakes in the 'sexing' must have been made because another family arrived in the girls' box, too. Another box was needed! Poor Dad! Meanwhile, Winnie and Bobbie had had yet another family, but we did not want to separate them, as they had been together for a long time, so we just removed the little ones as soon as they were old enough and left Winnie and Bobbie together.

'It's completely out of hand,' said Dad. 'I'm afraid we can't keep up. Some of these mice will have to go to the pet shop.'

He was sorry about this and thought that I would be upset. But I had realised that we could not go on like this, and as long as I could keep Winnie and Bobbie, I did not mind. I knew that they might have more babies, but we would send those to the pet shop when the time came. I think we took about 50 mice to the shop, and I earned money for the first time ever: a total of ten shillings.

Bobbie and Winnie did *not* have any more babies. They were getting too old, Dad said. I think they went on for a while, and I liked just having them without the worry of dozens of families of mice, but eventually they died—within a day of each other. I don't remember which went first, but I wrapped them in an old hankie of Dad's, put them in a glucose tin and had a very respectful funeral. Dad and Mum stood nearby as I put the tin into a hole that Dad had dug for me. I filled the hole and put a plant on top, together with a cross made of bits of wood.

I thought how nice of Dad and Mum to be there and not to tease me. I think they knew that I had been very fond of those mice.

The Salvage Competition

We had never come across the word 'salvage', but one day Miss Martin came into the classroom with a ball of string. She placed it on her desk, saying nothing.

We all said, 'Good morning, Miss Martin,' and sang our morning hymn.

Miss Martin said a brief prayer.

We were sure that she would tell us what the string was for then. But no.

We started our sums as usual but kept looking at the string on the desk, wondering if it was for a game or something like that. Our attention must have wandered because Miss Martin eventually said that we should stop what we were doing, as we were distracted and our work would be compromised. We had no idea what that meant, but we were very happy to stop doing sums.

At last she told us what this ball of string was for. There was to be a village Salvage Competition.

'What's that, Miss?' David was always the spokesman.

'Different groups are collecting anything useful for the war effort.'

'Like the Scrap Iron Drive, Miss?'

Miss Martin had not been at the school for the Scrap Iron Drive, so she was given a much-embellished version of that time.

Eventually, we were told that the scouts were collecting old clothes; the guides were to collect old sheets and pillowcases; and the school would collect waste paper.

We all groaned at this because most people used their old newspapers to light the fire, so we knew we wouldn't do well, but Miss Martin said that we must do our best. Once more, we were paired off and told to meet up on Saturday at the school. We had to measure out lengths of string to tie up bundles of paper and take about a dozen with each pair. So at last we knew what the ball of string was for . . .

This time, I had no bother at home at all because Mum remembered the Scrap Iron Drive. Sheila produced the old pram again, and we started at the village end of the road that we had been given as our 'patch'. We were amazed at how well we did! Thinking back, I realise that it was not all that surprising. Those were the days of no television, uncertain wireless information and the daily delivery of newspapers. Nearly everyone had a paper in order to keep up with the war news, and young boys made plenty of pocket money doing a paper round.

The pram was soon piled high with paper—nearly all newspaper, but some old letters and envelopes and a few posh magazines (we had a quick peek at these). We took one load back to school, making piles in the hallway, and then set off to do the other end of our road.

We trundled down a side lane to a very old, creepy-looking house and timidly knocked the door. A very, *very* old lady opened the door just a crack. She was extremely deaf, and it took us a long time to make her understand what we were doing. Finally, she drew back and opened the door wide. There, all along the hall and up the stairs, were piles and piles of papers! We just stared.

'Take them all,' she shouted, making us jump. She didn't know how loudly she spoke.

We looked at one another and then began to heave these bundles, already tied up, onto the pram. When it was full, we said we would come back for some more later. She smiled and nodded.

Back at school, we told Miss Martin, who was there to oversee the stacking of the piles. She said that she would send some of the others to help us when they returned, so there was a steady stream of children in and out of that house, gradually clearing the hall and the stairs. The old lady seemed delighted and kept nodding and smiling. She was a little bit scary because she had no teeth and her mouth looked huge when she smiled.

We had just about finished by four o'clock, when we were expected back at school for the last time, so Sheila and I went in to the room where the old lady was sitting knitting to say that we were going. We stopped and stared! Every wall of the room was almost hidden behind more and more bundles of old newspapers!

We jumped again as she shouted, 'You take these, too?'

We didn't know what to say. We were due back at school and the pram was full. We said that we would ask the teacher. She didn't understand us and looked cross, so we scuttled away.

Miss Martin listened to our tale and seemed to be deep in thought.

'I wonder if your daddy would take his car there, perhaps this evening, and you could load the trunk and bring it all back here in one trip.'

I was very proud to think that Miss Martin thought my father would help. Now I had to hope that he would.

'I will ask him,' I said.

I rushed home, clutching Miss Martin's phone number. Dad was intrigued by the sound of that 'batty old soul's' house and was glad to help.

Sheila and I went with Dad. At first, the old lady would not let Dad in, only opening the door a crack, as she had at first to us.

Then she recognised us and bellowed to us to come in. Dad heaved lots of the papers at a time into his big strong arms, while Sheila and I plodded patiently back and forth with as much as we could carry.

At last the room was empty of papers, but the walls and the floor were covered in cobwebs and dust. It looked as though nothing had been moved for years.

Dad shouted, 'Thank you,' and, 'Goodbye,' but the lady came outside after us.

'What about the rest?' she bellowed.

We stood still. More?

She turned to go in, shouting over her shoulder, 'In the shed.'

Dad looked at us and shrugged. We set off for an old shed in the overgrown garden.

Dad opened the door. 'Oh! My Lord!' he said.

You couldn't even get *into* the shed, there was so much paper.

'Oh no! No more. You've done enough!' Dad shut the door and went back to tell the lady that we couldn't take any more, but she had her wireless on so loudly that she didn't hear him hammering on the door.

The school won by a mile, having about ten times as much salvage as the Guides and Scouts. We didn't get a prize, but we didn't mind.

It had been an adventure.

The Scholarship

As 1943 loomed, I was eleven years old and approaching an event that not so much *changed* my life as determined its future direction more than anything else had since the death of my mother.

The examination to gain a scholarship to the Grammar school took place one bright June day. There had been no extra work, no homework; in fact, no real preparation at all. Our parents were scarcely aware that it was taking place except that the 'little ones' had the day off. Apart from this, I remember nothing of that day.

Today, children will be coached: they are probably very aware that much is riding on their performance, and parents may be as nervous as their offspring. Parental help with revision is normal, and a serious and rather tense atmosphere surrounds the preparations and the day itself. There is also a general expectation that most children will pass an exam.

In our time, very few passed the eleven-plus. Grammar schools were not large, so the questions had to be tailored to allow just a few to obtain this coveted scholarship. Those who failed went to secondary modern schools and often left at the age of fifteen.

After this most important but unremarkable day, several weeks went by without a thought about the exam. Then one morning after prayers, Miss Martin announced that there were three lucky children in the class. We were puzzled until she reminded us about the examination and told us that the results had arrived.

She gave the names of two other girls, then read out mine! I was amazed. I had not given it a thought, either to assume that I would not pass or that I might. But the fact that the other two girls were acknowledged to be 'clever' made it most surprising to me that my name had been announced, too.

I don't think we even got a clap before the lesson went ahead as usual. There were no concessions, acknowledgements or celebrations. It was just a normal day. But I was seething with excitement, pride and amazement and couldn't wait for the end of the afternoon.

I ran most of the way home: out of the playground, through the village, down the hill along by the river, and burst into the kitchen.

'I've got the scholarship, Mum!'

She was standing with her back to me. Without turning, she said, 'Hah! You? You never have!'

I was numb. Had I been a bath full of water, it would have been like pulling the plug.

In a tiny, lifeless voice, I said, 'I have, Mum.'

She gave a kind of laugh. 'No, you haven't,' she said again, then went back to whatever she was doing.

'I have, Mum.'

'No, you haven't. You are not clever enough for anything like that.'

I persisted. 'Three of us. Elaine, Barbara and me.'

Then she looked round and peered at me. She took a big breath. 'Are you sure? How do you know?'

'Miss Martin announced it at prayers this morning. Elaine, Barbara and me.'

'She definitely said you, did she?'

'Yes, Mum.' There was no fun in it anymore. I was too close to tears to care much now. If she didn't believe me . . . well.

Mum started to wipe her hands and finally *really* looked at me.

'Well, if you are really sure, we had better ring your dad, I suppose.' She *still* did not seem happy.

There was an extension from the house to the Works. The phone was on a hook on the wall, and I had only just grown tall enough to reach it and the horn-shaped speaker, which was even higher.

She turned the little handle to make the phone ring at the Works. When Dad answered, she said, rather slowly and still doubtfully, 'Julia has something to tell you.'

I took the phone and told him the news, but I couldn't sound excited any more. He was amazed and delighted and did not seem to doubt me.

'You don't sound very excited about it,' he said.

My pride and relief were bringing the excitement back, though, and I was so thrilled when he said that he would come home right away. By the time he arrived, Mum had the tea ready, and the three of us sat down round the table together. This rarely happened except for Sunday dinner. They sat looking at me. Mum still seemed slightly puzzled, but Dad was very pleased and smiled and smiled at me. They had a doubting look about them, as though they could still hardly believe that this child before them, whom they had obviously thought to be of minimal intelligence, must actually have some brains.

Many, many years later I encountered the same look from a member of the family when I had a book published. That look is certainly not flattering, but, as a child, I just glowed under their attention, and I was beginning to realise that at last I might have shown that I was worth . . . something. I didn't know exactly what—but I was glad that they were pleased and impressed.

The Country Nurse Remembers

All the details about the school itself and the arrangements for train travel and the worry about coupons for the uniform would come later.

For now, I was in a happy bubble.

The First Day

I was sick five times in the night and twice in the hedge on the way to the train on the first morning of my first term at the City of Bath Girls' Grammar School, to give it its full name.

I was not ill, just so very nervous. I had now been at the same small school of about forty children for five years and had become used to the lessons, the village and the children. Now I was off to a large school of about four hundred girls, who would be coming from the city itself and many villages all around. I would be in year one among the youngest girls in the school.

I was the first on the station platform—this was always to be the case, as Mum made me leave home very early—and I sat shivering with nerves. I had never been on a train without Mum. I was very conscious that the eczema on my legs had worsened, and I knew that the girls would notice it and might think, like the village children, that it was catching. I was also worrying about the fact that all new girls had to see the headmistress on their first day to be interviewed, whatever that meant. It sounded frightening.

I was the only new girl from the village, after all. Barbara's parents had decided to send her to the secondary modern school, although she had won a scholarship. No one could understand this decision at first, but we thought it must be because she wanted to be with her older sister at the school. Elaine's parents used the scholarship to send her to a posh school somewhere, so she was not with me, either.

The school itself looked enormous to me. It had been a huge private house many, many years ago when the school was created. Extension after extension had been built, so that it now had two gyms, a hall with a stage, many classrooms, an art block, two science labs, shower rooms, a library and so on. There were four tennis courts and extensive grounds. I thought it was lovely, but frighteningly large. I was sure I would get lost! Some of the girls had their mothers with them, but they were sent away after we went in.

The new girls lined up outside the headmistress's study (I was intrigued—I had never been in a study before), and we had to wait for the light over the door to change from red to green before we could go in.

I knocked and Miss Prestige said, 'Come in!'

'You do not need to knock,' she continued. 'You just wait for the light to change.'

I felt like an idiot because I had knocked instinctively—I still had to announce my arrival this way before entering any room at home. But I could not tell her that! She was very nice, with a quiet, very precise voice, and she peered short-sightedly at me through her pebble glasses. She hoped I would work hard and be happy in the school. She also said that my mother had rung to say that I had been so very sick, and she asked if I was better now.

'Yes, thank you,' I said, and that was probably the last time I spoke to her for about two years. She seemed kind but very remote.

I liked the school, especially the art block, the gym and the library. As first years, we were only allowed in the library under supervision, but I could not believe my eyes when I saw the number of books there. I did not know that there were that many books in the world! Later, I loved to sit in the seats in the little dormer-type windows and read, read and read.

The first year was divided into three classes: L, B and C. I was astonished to find that I was in the top class, which was 'L', for the Latin class. We were presumed to be bright enough to learn Latin, and, while I was never brilliant at it, I have always been glad that I studied it. Suddenly, I was to learn English language and English literature: we had only ever done reading and writing at the village school!

French, history, geography and art, all of which I loved, were on the curriculum, as was science, which I didn't like at all. Biology became a favourite and best of all was gym: *real* gym in a wonderful gymnasium. I was surprised that Scripture was taught in a classroom and not in a church. The three sorts of maths were a nightmare, and domestic science, which included sewing, caused a lot of trouble at home. As Mum had been a dressmaker, she insisted that the way I was being taught some sewing techniques was wrong and that I should do certain things her way. I spent many an early morning on the station, trying to unpick whatever I had done at home Mum's way and redoing it to suit the rather booming DS mistress. Unsurprisingly, I did not get good marks.

It was all overwhelming at first, but gradually I began to find my way around, and I made friends with a girl called June, who seemed to come from a very strict home, as I did. We did not talk about it, but we formed an instinctive bond, which lasted until we left the school.

I settled in to the routine: one could do nothing else. There was strict discipline based on naming and shaming, and being made to stand in the corridor, or miss games or—horror of horrors—being sent to the headmistress. Over the years, I spent some time standing in corridors (usually for talking in class); I also missed one games lesson. But I managed to avoid being sent to the headmistress.

Worse still, for me, was the threat of a letter to my parents. Luckily, the only one that got sent home to Mum was asking her not to send me to school with a streaming cold again. This had happened several times, and I had just been sent back home. There were few trains in the middle of the day, so I would just have to wait on the station; sometimes, when I got home, Mum was not there, and so I had to sit in the greenhouse to wait for her. Mum was always very cross when she found me back home and seemed to think that it was my fault. I could never understand it.

The emphasis at school was on good academic work, respect for staff and a realisation that we were 'young ladies'. This was most important. Anything rough or the slightest bit uncouth was not tolerated. And, indeed, there *was* great respect for the staff, amounting, in several cases, to abject fear. One mistress had piercing blue eyes, and, as she was a maths teacher, I was always falling foul of her. I was no good at maths anyway, but when in her presence I was a nervous wreck. I think she left under some sort of cloud; a scandal, we believed. It was all very intriguing.

In among all these new experiences I also felt a sense of freedom. I was away from home for most of each day, with interesting girls and learning new things. I was surprised to find that the staff and girls had opinions about things that were different from Mum and Dad's, and I listened with amazement to snippets of conversation among them. Many of the girls were only my age, so how did they know all these things?

At first, Mum and Dad were genuinely interested in the school and the lessons, and I seemed to have tea with them more often in order to tell them all about it. When I told them that I was in the top class of the year, they believed me straight away and seemed pleased.

Although I would not have realised it, this was the beginning of the next phase of my childhood. There had been the 'before time', which I still thought about sometimes with nostalgia; the muddled time after Mummy's death; then the settled time in the village school; and now the opening up of the academic world. Mum's strict control was still there, of course, and I was frequently very miserable, but when I was at school I often managed to forget the problems at home.

The years gradually passed.

I did well in piano and singing. The piano playing was not more than average, but the singing was evidently good. After a concert in the third year, the head of music said that I should take it up, meaning have singing lessons with a view to a career in music. Mum and Dad would not hear of it. I should have a 'proper job' when I left, not some silly singing stuff, they said. Nothing more was said about it. We did not have careers information nor were we told about grants for further education; I did not know that there were such things, and I suppose that Mum and Dad didn't, either.

I was also quite good at hockey. I was average to small and fast on my feet, so the forward line suited me, and I was soon playing for my junior house team. The games mistress said that I should play in the *school* junior team, but the matches took place on Saturdays, so I had to ask Mum and Dad.

'No,' said Mum. 'You would be away all Saturday morning, which is when you do the bedrooms and the sitting room, and suppose we wanted to go out?'

So that was that.

I wanted to be a Girl Guide too, but that would have interrupted one evening a week and some days in the holidays, so that was out, as well.

The Country Nurse Remembers

At school, I became interested in medical matters. I found biology, which included the anatomy and physiology of the human body, fascinating, and by the time I was about 13 or 14, I had decided that I wanted to become a doctor. No one else in the class seemed to know what they wanted to do, so I kept quiet for a long time. I knew it might mean spending a long time training and I realised that this would cost money, so I was not surprised when I eventually broached the subject at home that I was told it might not be possible. Mum said she didn't think I would be clever enough anyway, but Dad said they would 'make the sacrifice' if necessary.

I began to be afraid that I would have to be 'kept' by them, and that would mean that I would have to ask for everything and there would be no freedom from Mum's domination. I did not think it through in quite such a clear-cut way, but the general feeling was there that I would be 'beholden'—that was a word I had heard and understood.

So, very early in my school life, I decided to go for second best. Nursing. I knew that I would live away from home, in a nurses' hostel, and be paid (just) for my work and for the intermittent college times, and that it only took three years to become qualified.

That would be a 'proper job', which would please Mum and Dad, and they wouldn't have to 'keep' me. Very importantly, it also meant I would be able to leave home. So I told them, and everyone, that I was going to be a nurse.

They were delighted; Grandma and Grandpa thought it was a very hard job to choose, and Grandma S. said she could not imagine having to touch ill people. Granddad S. said it was a calling. It wasn't really because I had worked it all out, but I did want to help sick people, and this was the nearest thing to being a doctor.

The immediate effect of this decision was that I was allowed to join the St John Ambulance's Junior Brigade. Although this meant doing first-aid training once a week in the evening and going out with the ambulance to various functions, like point-to-point races on a Saturday sometimes, I was allowed to do this, as it would be useful later on and, as I was told, I could always do the bedrooms on Sunday.

It was good fun, and I was learning a lot. However, at the races I was far more upset when the horses were hurt than the jockeys. Was this the way a nurse should feel? Probably not. What about being a vet instead, I asked myself?

I mentioned this in passing to Mum, who was horrified that I should even think about changing my mind. It had only been a very vague idea, but Mum said that once I had made up my mind, I must stick to it. So I did. What a mouse I was!

The Pictures

There had been little bombing in the South-West for some months now, and we had stopped sleeping in the shelter altogether. It was kept ready, however, for as Dad said, 'You never know.' We had air-raid practice in school, but where we went for shelter, I do not remember. We carried our gas masks, were reminded by notices in the trains that 'careless talk costs lives' and wore our uniform clothes until they were ridiculously short and tight—new ones took so many coupons. Prayers were said in the daily assembly for the military personnel and all others suffering the consequences of war, but it all sounded very formal and unreal. Here, there were no boys to give their enthusiastic and improbable interpretation of events.

I think we were desensitised by now. There were so many deaths in the fields of conflict, so much suffering in the occupied countries and so many ships sunk that our minds ceased to take it all in. We were discouraged from talking about the war at school because the fathers of many of the girls were in the forces. From time to time, a girl would be called out of class to be told that her father had been killed, captured or wounded. The child concerned would be away from school for a week or so, and we would all be told to be especially nice to her when she returned. We *were* sorry—we were not monsters—but there was so much of it all that we soon concentrated once more on our own affairs.

We were aware, however, of the arrival of the American GIs. It was long after the war that I was told that 'GI' meant 'Government Issue'. I wonder if the handsome, swaggering Americans themselves knew this. I can't imagine that they would have been impressed!

Many Americans were billeted in and around Bath. America had joined the war after the bombing of Pearl Harbor in 1941, but on the whole I was not aware of their presence in England until they appeared in their dozens in Bath. They were a source of great worry to mothers of the women who fell for these glamorous young men in their smart uniforms, who were known to have plenty of money, cigarettes and silk stockings and an eye for the girls. The saying sprang up that they were 'over-paid, over-sexed and over here'!

Bath was still in a poor state, with damaged buildings, big open spaces where houses had stood and piles of rubble where buddleia bushes and foxgloves flourished. Buddleia, although beautiful, still reminds me of devastation.

I was in my second year when the country started to become more hopeful that the war could be brought to an end fairly soon. An air of excitement was felt, and people spoke of the invasion of Germany as a real possibility. It was rumoured that various main roads were closed some nights to ordinary traffic (there wasn't much anyway) for troop movements towards the south coast, ready to cross the Channel, but everything was hush-hush.

At about this time, Mum and Dad decided we would start going to the pictures on Friday evenings. So for the first time, aged about twelve, I went to the pictures with them. I don't remember the main film at all, but I remember the Pathé News. Suddenly, I was seeing soldiers, aircraft, ships, Mr. Churchill and much more. A voice told us of the terrible cruelty of the Germans. Then we were seeing Japanese soldiers with guns standing over thin men who were digging and building a road. I watched as the police, here at home, arrested someone for selling things on the black market, and I saw a group of men rebuilding a bomb-damaged house. It was all so amazing!

I realised that, in time, I might be able to join in some of the chatter among the girls at school: they had been going to the pictures regularly and knew all about film stars with wonderful hair and clothes and a place called Hollywood, where the films were made and everyone was rich and lived in enormous houses and walked around all day in their bathing costumes. At least that is the way it seemed to me. Just as television opened up the post-war world to ordinary people, so the cinema was doing the same for the quiet corners of wartime Britain. The light and glamour of the American films, with their unlikely stories, the glimpses into a world without black-out, shortages, gas masks and bombs, were just what everyone needed to raise their spirits, Dad told me.

Although I was far too young to appreciate them, the dance halls, with their noisy bands and lively tunes, were another diversion. Everyone needed some light-hearted entertainment to banish the gloom of war-torn Britain.

I loved the pictures except for two things. The cinema was always blue with smoke from the hundreds of cigarettes that were being smoked, and my eyes streamed. The other thing was the plush seats! The bristly surface of the seat hurt and irritated the eczema on the back of my knees so that I kept trying to ease the pain by sitting forward so that my knees were beyond the edge of the seat. Mum kept telling me to stop fidgeting and sit back. Even Dad realised that it was painful for me, but when he pointed this out to Mum she just said, 'If she sits still, it will be all right.' Of course, it wasn't, so Dad gave me his soft hankie to put behind my knees.

Soon I would be taken to the doctor and given some proper ointment, and while it did not cure the eczema, it soothed the pain and itching a bit.

The patches behind my ears were a problem at school, being on show all the time because of my short hair. I was intensely miserable about this, as, apart from the embarrassment of the eczema, I was the only girl in the entire school with hair so short and straight. Hair was being worn at shoulder length or long in plaits at that time.

For the first, but not the last, time, I became devious. I told Mum that the teachers thought that the cut ends of my hair were irritating my skin and making it raw (it was actually what *I* wondered) and that I ought to grow my hair so that the ends were below the back of my ears. I got myself in knots with this lie, but it worked. A very grudging Mum eventually agreed. It did help, and what a difference this apparently minor change made to my life.

Another lie followed because of Mum's insistence that I should wear the thick grey winter uniform stockings all through the summer, as well. This was awful. Everyone wore white ankle socks in the summer. The gym mistress asked me if I was going to wear these stockings all the summer. I said that I was. Why did I not tell her that I hated the idea and that Mum made me? Like everything else, I seemed to protect Mum from ridicule. Was I self-conscious maybe and didn't want people to know about my situation at home? I don't know, even now. I told Mum that the teacher had said that I must not wear the stockings in the summer because it was very bad for me. She *had* said that it was bad for me, but I added the rest.

Another lie that I told concerned the showers. I loved the showers (no one had showers at home; only baths), but occasionally I was afraid that I might have bruises on the tops of my legs, so I didn't want to undress. We were only excused a shower if it was 'that time of the month', so I sometimes pretended to the gym mistress that it was, when it wasn't. No one ever questioned this, as it was considered a very private and delicate matter.

The Country Nurse Remembers

All these personal things mattered hugely, even though the world around me was tearing itself apart in the war. How selfish we were at that age.

I was just entering my teens, but the term 'teenager' had not been coined. We were children until we were adults. There was no in-between.

Legally you were an adult at twenty-one, when you 'came of age' and got 'the key of the door', although many youngsters had jobs from about fifteen or went to college at eighteen. In spite of this, most were still under the care and control of their parents until they were about twenty.

How very different things are now.

'Peace in Our Time'

It seems extraordinary to me that I should be writing about the end of the war in Europe today, the 11th of November at roughly eleven a.m. I had not planned the progress of my tale to coincide with this iconic day at all, I just happened to arrive at that momentous event on this year's Armistice Day.

Of the actual end of the war I remember absolutely nothing. No announcement in school—though there must have been one—no jubilation at home, no street party or service of thanksgiving; nothing! I was only seven when the war had started, but I remember exactly where I was and what was said by my father and how he looked that day. I was thirteen now, and yet I remember nothing at all about such a joyous occasion as the end of this long, grim war.

Gradually the lights went on, signposts were reinstated, air-raid shelters were demolished or turned into garden sheds, men came home and many were demobbed. The Americans started to go home too, some taking with them an English wife: a 'GI Bride'. Large numbers of people were still homeless as a result of earlier bombing, so cheap houses were quickly built. They were called prefabs and were only meant to last for ten years, but some would still be occupied more than fifty years later. Work started on the restoration of Bath Abbey and some of the other historic buildings in the city. Excavation began again on the Roman Baths, while the trains and buses no longer carried the warnings about careless talk or exhortations to dig for victory.

But all this took a long time: materials were still in short supply, factories had to be restructured towards their original function after making munitions and many skilled workers had been lost. Rationing was expected to ease, but it actually got much tighter as 'we' were helping to feed the starving in Europe; and, with so much of our merchant shipping lost, overseas goods were still virtually unavailable. As children, we could not really understand all this and rather thought that this wonderful victory would mean a return to normality immediately. Mind you, many of us were too young to remember what 'normality' had been like anyway.

At the pictures, I saw the London celebrations, with all their pomp and flag waving, but I also realised that whatever Bath and Bristol had suffered in the bombing, it was nothing like the devastation that Londoners had experienced and which I now saw, stretching away behind the bands and parades and all the jubilation. At last, I was beginning to think outside our own corner of England.

A few days later, what I saw on the cinema screen was to have a profound effect on me for a very, very long time.

Friday came. Once more, I do not remember the main film, but, even now, all these decades later, I can see the horrendous images on the screen on the Pathé News.

Images of the victory celebrations were shown, and then the music went silent and the cinema manager came on to the stage in front of the screen. He said that they had been told to warn people that they were about to see upsetting pictures from a concentration camp that the British troops had liberated during the invasion of Germany. The authorities had advised that these were not suitable for children, so there were staff available to take children out to the foyer and look after them there. He disappeared, and streams of children started to pass on their way out.

Mum said to Dad, 'Should Julia go out, then?'

After a moment, Dad said, 'No, I want her to see this and remember . . . '

So I stayed.

Pictures were shown of the conditions in an infamous concentration camp, the name of which I cannot bring myself to write even now. A group of British officials were being taken round this terrible place, accompanied by the Pathé cameras.

There were piles of bodies everywhere, some mutilated, some burnt, all nearly naked and so thin that they were like skeletons. Among them were small children's bodies. The officials were shown the instruments of torture, hammers and knives, that had been used on the people, then the ovens in which they were burnt, whether alive or dead, I have never known. A commentator said, 'The living walked about among the dead.'

Then there was some hazy footage taken by the first soldiers to enter, and it showed some living people sitting, slumped against a wall, so thin that they could scarcely sit and again almost naked. Then we saw the fat, brutal-looking German commandant, being arrested. We saw the shocked and horrified faces of the liberating troops. There was more, but I closed my eyes at that stage and held my breath to prevent myself from being sick.

From that evening onwards, for about twelve months, I could scarcely sleep for the horror of the pictures in my mind. When I did fall asleep, I dreamed that the bodies rose from the ground and walked towards me. In the day, I kept seeing images of flames in those ovens and the dead bodies of the children, just thrown into a heap. I seemed to scream in my mind.

I could not bear to be alone because I thought of that place all the time, and I could not bear to be with people in case they spoke about it. Many did, as the shock waves of the discovery of such appalling atrocities spread through the country. I walked away from groups of girls at school if there was the slightest chance that they might speak of it; I skipped biology one day because we were going to study the effects of starvation on the human body, and I guessed that the atrocities would be discussed.

I could not eat, my marks slipped at school and my friends took me to task for being 'peculiar'. I shrugged it off with a sort of bravado, pretending that there was nothing wrong. I could not turn to anyone for help, as that would have meant talking about it. In any case, it would not have occurred to me that I *could* be helped. Some teachers asked if I was all right and, of course, I said yes, but all the time the terrible images of what I had seen went on and on in my head, in my chest, it seemed, and in my tummy.

Tummy ache and 'bilious attacks' were the norm, but on two occasions they were so bad that I had to stay home from school. With this and my poorer marks, Mum said that I should keep to school more. Dad stuck up for me, saying that it was not my fault. I did not think at the time that this was ironic, as it was really *his* fault for making me watch that newsreel. That realisation came years later.

I no longer wanted to go to the pictures in case there was something else like that in the news, but Mum and Dad insisted that I go with them. I couldn't tell them why I didn't want to go. They noticed nothing specific, except that Mum said I was slower than usual at doing the bedrooms and Aunt Lizzy thought I was paler than ever. She was wise enough not to say this to Mum this time.

Dad was very distressed by the cruelty at the time, but it did not occur to him that I might be, too. If it had, he would have wanted to talk me out of it; and I couldn't have that, so I tried not to be with him very much. It was as well that he did not notice this, either. So my anxiety went on for months and months.

I tried to think how to tell Mum and Dad that I no longer wanted to be a nurse, without telling them why. I might have to see and cope with the results of cruelty or tend sick little children. I knew that I couldn't do that. I worried and worried about this, but then another emotion took over. Guilt! Guilt that I was alive and they were dead. Guilt that I was often miserable at home, but at least I *had* a home. Guilt that I was afraid to be a nurse. I was only twelve or thirteen so I don't think I itemised these feelings quite like this, but that was generally how I felt.

But gradually I decided that I would feel less guilty if I *did* become a nurse. I could help children—not those poor children, they had gone forever, but sick children in hospitals. So I wanted to be a nurse again, this time with a more altruistic motive than just wanting to leave home!

One of the officials who had inspected the concentration camp was the MP for our area and sometime in the following few months she committed suicide. I do not remember if the reason was discovered or reported, but in my young mind I *knew*, without a doubt, that she was suffering because of all the terrible sights she had seen and that she couldn't live with those memories. I was totally convinced of this, reasoning that I had only seen it on the screen: how much worse it must have been for her to have actually been there.

Until that time, I had been sure that God had been on our side—we had been told often enough—but now I wondered. How could He have let these awful things happen before He helped us to win the war? The only way I could deal with that thought was to believe that the Devil had been at work.

I do not talk of that time, but it slowly passed as everything does.

The following year I was thankful that I had a lot of *good* things to think about.

Growing Up

Great News

I was in the 'other room' one day when Mum called from the dining room. I knocked the door, but there was no answer. So I knocked again. Dad's voice sounded impatient when he said, 'Oh, do come in!' I entered just as Mum came in from the kitchen.

'For goodness sake, Mildred,' he said, 'why on earth the child has to knock on doors all the time, I don't know. We will have no more of it!'

Mum pursed her lips. 'Oh well,' she said. 'Sit down. We want to tell you something.'

I sat at the table opposite Dad. Mum was to my left.

Dad said, 'Who do you think is coming to live with us?'

I immediately answered, 'Auntie Jinny?' (Wishful thinking!)

They looked taken aback, and then Dad said, 'No, not Auntie Jinny or anyone like that. It will be a brother or sister for you.'

I went hot and cold. I knew exactly what this meant and I could feel the excitement welling up inside me, but I did not dare to say what I thought in case it was wrong. It would have been so embarrassing! So I just looked at Dad and then at Mum and said nothing.

'Well, can't you think?' said Mum.

'Um . . . is it . . . are you going to have a baby?' I was so afraid that somehow I was wrong and they would hoot with laughter, but they both smiled.

'That's right.'

I took a big breath: 'Oh, I'm so glad. When?'

'Oh, a while yet. May. We told you first. Now we shall tell Grandma and Granddad S. and Grandma and Grandpa and Aunt Lizzy.

'Can I come too, when you tell them?' I wanted to be part of the excitement. I thought everyone would be as thrilled as I was. But they were all a bit worried at first because Mum was now thirty-seven and this was considered a bit old to have a *first* baby, although many women had subsequent babies into their late forties.

Dad was a bit quiet about it sometimes, and Mum said it was because *my* mother had died when she'd had a baby, and for the first time Mum talked a little about my mother. I was astonished and slightly apprehensive, and I wondered what she was going to say.

She told me that I had been a Caesar birth. I had an idea that this meant that my mother had needed to have the baby taken out in an operation rather than the 'natural' way. The natural way was still a bit amazing to me, as I found it difficult to imagine that 'things' could stretch to make room for a baby to get through. Mum went on to say that the doctors had advised my mother not to have any more babies. This was quite usual, as Caesarean operations were much more risky then than they are now. However, my mother had so wanted another baby that the doctors had finally said that she would be all right so long as she had it by another Caesarean section rather than trying to have it naturally. (I don't think anyone has ever known why she could not give birth in the usual way.)

So she went off to hospital to have the baby, and the operation was performed. My mother actually died from septicaemia *after* the birth rather than from the birth itself. Her little daughter died too, perhaps of septicaemia; no one seemed to know. There were no antibiotics generally available in 1938, although they had been discovered. Septicaemia is easily cured these days.

Mum said that Dad was worried that it could all happen again. This was a bit silly, but understandable, as he had lost one wife in childbirth, but Mum was a much more robust sort of person and he was worrying unnecessarily.

'I thought you ought to know,' Mum said, after she had shared these details with me.

I thanked her for telling me, and, for the first time, I felt that there might be a sort of bond because I was another female in a world where pregnancy and childbirth were not readily discussed—and certainly not with men—and because I was obviously so happy about the coming baby: *her* baby.

There was no chance of buying lots of baby clothes and equipment in austere, post-war Britain, so Mum made clothes and cut up towels to make nappies. Some coupons were issued to pregnant mums, but they did not go far, only buying a very few napkins and cot sheets. Disposable nappies were unheard of. Dad bought a second-hand cot, which he painted white, a carrycot and a funny little folding pram to fit onto the back seat of the car.

I was told not to tell the girls at school. Why, I wondered?

But I did tell them. I couldn't keep such a wonderful piece of news to myself.

People rarely used the words 'pregnant' and 'pregnancy'. One was 'expecting' or even 'in an interesting condition', although that term was dying out. A mother still stayed in bed for about two weeks after having a baby, the 'lying in' period. Many women had their babies at home, as the NHS did not appear until 1948 and nursing home care was very expensive. Dad insisted that Mum should not have the baby at home and booked a local place for her straight away. It was a bright, airy house with only four single rooms and a delivery room. Mrs. Gill, a retired hospital matron, owned and ran the 'home', with the help of several nurses, while the local doctor visited regularly and was always on call. It was all very relaxed and civilised, unlike the frenetic atmosphere of modern maternity hospitals, now dealing with an ever-increasing number of births.

So life and school went on while we waited for the great event. Many of the girls at school who had brothers and sisters could not understand why I was so excited, but I must have had an over-active maternal instinct, as I could think of little else. This might have been a blessing, as the horrors that had haunted me for so many months were gradually replaced by thoughts of the baby; I was still unable to speak about those things, but I no longer had so many nightmares, or day-mares, and I could make a positive effort to think of other things.

My hair was growing and the eczema behind my ears had almost gone, I was getting better marks again at school and doing well in music and biology. I seemed to have caught the attention of the English mistress, Miss Pence (nickname Penny, of course). She commended my story writing and my oral work, so that I glowed with pride.

I was in the gym team for gym displays—I have forgotten why we had displays or what they achieved—and I was doing well at swimming. So I felt happier than I had for a long time and seemed to be fitting in with more of the girls now.

I had passed several piano exams and enjoyed playing, but Mum would not allow me to do anything except practice my scales—I so wanted to have fun on the piano, making up tunes. Practising scales was boring, so as soon as I started to get a lot of homework, I asked if I could give up the lessons. Later I regret-ted this decision, but I did not get home from school until after five, *if* the train was on time, and I was still expected to be in bed by about seven, so there really was very little time for anything other than homework in the week. Saturday was chores day or St. John Ambulance, and Sunday was more chores and getting things ready for Monday.

About this time Mum and Dad started to play bridge with some neighbours on Friday evenings. I had to go as well, and sit nearby and read. I loved reading, but there I had to sit bolt upright all evening, with my feet neatly together and the book held by both hands in front of my face. No leaning back in the chair, no easing of legs or feet, or resting of arms. Mum's stern eye was on me, and if I had a foot in the wrong place, her finger would flick an instruction as she sat at the table with her fan of cards. I got very tired and at moments like those was very aware of how extreme some of Mum's rules were. I said nothing, but I was beginning to think that perhaps she was not always right.

At least Mrs. Tanner gave me a cup of tea and a biscuit when they all paused for refreshments.

Most of Dad's 'chaps' had returned from the war and were only too happy to have a job to go to, so Dad had a little more time to spare. He suddenly realised that I had been able to swim for some time now, and, being a strong swimmer himself, he decided to take me to the baths occasionally. We had races. For just a couple of lengths I could beat him, but if we tried longer races, he was always well ahead. I loved diving, but Dad would not try it. Mum hated the water, and, even if she had not been pregnant, she would not have joined us. It was nice to have Dad to myself and we had fun. I was still very much a child, even at fourteen.

Dad always needed a hobby—a practical one. He decided that future holidays with a new baby would be difficult (children were not welcomed in hotels and restaurants as they are now), so he began to build a caravan. Caravans and caravan sites were very new, and to actually build your own caravan was considered odd but enterprising. Dad asked me if I would like to help him in the holidays and *of course* I said yes. I was delighted, and Mum seemed happier for me to be with Dad more now, whereas she had always found reasons why I should not help him in the garden, with the car, cleaning out the chickens and so on. I liked all these outside jobs, especially when I worked with Dad. As I have said: I should have been a boy.

Now, perhaps with her own baby coming, she was more inclined to let Dad spend more time with me. We worked very hard on that caravan, which I thought was marvellous, although it had none of the amenities that modern commercially manufactured ones do. We had several holidays in it until eventually Dad sold it. Some fifty years later, it was seen to be still in use—but only as a chicken house!

Added to the excitement of the coming brother or sister, I had a cautious feeling that life, in general, was getting better.

Robert

It wasn't long before May arrived. I had been sent to stay with Grandma S. in Bath while Mum was in the nursing home. I think I must have been at school when the baby came because Grandma told me when I got in for tea. Dad came later, wreathed in smiles and very relieved—he had been worried for days. He said that he was going to see Mum that evening and that he would take me the next day, as it was Saturday. Husbands did not stay with their wives for the birth of their children in those times and would have been shocked to the core to think that a man would do such a thing. Childbirth was very much a female-only time.

I finally saw my baby brother at three p.m. on Saturday. I thought he was gorgeous, and I loved him on the spot. I was allowed to cuddle him, but when he began to scream a nurse took him away. Mum looked a bit flushed but very proud, while Dad was just relieved that it was all over.

Previously, I had been given the immense privilege of choosing the baby's name. Margaret was my choice for a girl and Robert for a boy. I felt very honoured to have named him—it made me feel part of the event, and I kept telling him his name as I held him.

When Mum and Robert came home, I couldn't wait to help with him, dress him, take him out in his pram and most of all cuddle him. Mum stuck rigidly to the current thinking, which was to feed four-hourly exactly and not to pick the child up every time he cried unless there was something wrong, like wind. I hated to hear him cry and often got into trouble for pretending that he had wind so that I could pick him up. But he got used to Mum's routine fairly quickly and was a good baby.

When he was about three months old, we went to see Auntie Jinny. I think Dad, who was very fond of her, wanted her to see the baby. I did not have as much time with Auntie on my own as I had on previous occasions, but I loved showing Robert off to all her neighbours in the back gardens of the row of cottages.

However, one day we were by ourselves, sitting in the sun. Mum was resting and I had Robert on my lap.

'You are growing up,' Auntie said. 'I can't call you "little one" any more. You are taller than I am now.' She paused. 'Are you happy?'

I always tried to be truthful with Auntie. 'Sometimes, Auntie,' I said. 'School is all right . . . I have some nice friends . . . '

Auntie sighed, and, in a dreamy voice, she murmured, 'If only dear Phyll had lived!' Again, she paused. 'You look like her, you know.'

I wanted to cry, but I just hugged Robert and tried to smile at Auntie.

'You are as fond of that baby as if he were your own,' she said. 'I believe you know now how your dear mother loved you. It was the same, only much, much more.'

I realised then how wonderful my mother's love must have been because I could not imagine being able to feel any *more* love than I did for baby Robert.

But Auntie Jinny was always right about these things.

Last Days of School

At home, I was still a child, under strict supervision at all times, allowed no opinions of my own, no likes or dislikes that were not Mum's likes or dislikes, no freedom to come and go, no friends allowed in the house, no choice in clothes and very little in anything else (except Robert's name).

At school, I had received a good academic education, fitting me more than adequately for my chosen career, but socially I was totally unprepared for entry into the big, wide adult world of work and independence. School had instilled in us respect for authority and taught us how to conduct ourselves with decorum and the need to remember at all times that we were 'young ladies'. Parents were expected to ready girls for whatever career they would pursue or place in society they would fill, as they or the child saw it. This was often subject to the existing place in society of the family as a whole. For instance, I had problems making Mum and Dad, who both had regional accents, understand that I was only trying to speak properly rather than 'getting above myself' or being 'haughty'. Many children had to fight against their parents' ideas of some sort of preordained 'place' in society, which they would inevitably fill. This sounds incredibly old-fashioned, but it was still an attitude that persisted for some time after the war in rural areas, where change was not welcomed and new ideas were slow to be accepted.

Another more subtle change was happening to me at home. I had become more and more convinced that, so far as Mum was concerned, I had never stopped being 'the problem'. During the war years, there had been so much to think about and worry about and, on the whole, I had been useful and fitted in, so Mum had accepted me as part of the family. Now the war, with all its problems, was over. I was growing up and would be leaving soon and there was Robert.

Mum was not a 'lovey-dovey' mother to Robert, but she obviously loved her son very much. Rather than feeling any jealousy, I was very glad to know that he would have a better time than I had enjoyed. I realised that this was the family structure that Mum must always have longed for—Dad, Mum and their baby. I felt outside this; the one that did not fit into this picture. It was, perhaps, surprising that I didn't really mind. I suppose I had always known somehow that Mum resented having to look after me and that Dad had never noticed, so it was not a new scenario; it just seemed more obvious now. I didn't blame anyone. What would have been the point? It was just the way it was.

But at school I had found my place among the girls. I had always had my friend June, but, oddly, we never exchanged confidences and neither ever visited the other's home. She was a strong, solitary character, whereas I needed other people, so my circle of friends had grown.

Also I discovered boys. Or perhaps boys discovered me!

The single exception to the social restrictions imposed from home was to allow me to learn ballroom dancing! We combined with the Bath Boys School, our twin school, for some lessons, and one of the teachers involved started the Friday Socials. They took place in the boy's school hall from about 6:30 to 9:30 p.m., the first half consisting of instruction in the waltz, foxtrot, quick-step, samba, rumba, tango, Viennese waltz and some fun dances. The second half was when the boys, overcoming their shyness, asked the girls to dance. A 'Lady's choice' was always included.

Luckily, a letter had been sent to all the parents of senior girls (aged sixteen to eighteen), announcing the formation of these classes. The mistress concerned had made the letter most persuasive, and Mum fell for it. I was amazed. She said that she had liked dancing, so she thought I would enjoy it, too. So, at seventeen, I began for the first time to get a little pocket money to cover the cost of the classes. I started to enjoy the company of boys.

One very serious and gentle boy started to ask me to dance more often than any other, and he eventually flattered but horrified me by asking me to go to the pictures with him. I wanted to go, and I said I would ask Mum. But it was *Dad* who was against it.

'Oh no,' he said. 'That's too much like courting.'

Even then this was a very old-fashioned term.

'Bring him to tea,' Mum suggested.

I was aghast! He would see what a child I really was.

When Gordon came, he was very polite, if a little bemused, and was approved. We went to the pictures once or twice, and then he just gently faded from the picture. My one romance was over before it had begun. My one romance? There had been another. I had been all of eight years old when a small boy blushingly gave me *two* birthday cards because he could not afford a present, he said.

Mock school-leaving examinations were held and were quite difficult, so my marks were only average. But in the real ones some six months later I did very well—and even Mum was impressed. I think Dad had begun to realise that I had a few brains after all and was no longer surprised if I achieved good marks.

I did not think about my mother quite so often now, but somewhere in my mind was a little space kept only for her. Now, I wondered if she might know that I had done well at school. Had I been able to ask Auntie Jinny, she would have said, 'Of course she knows!' Auntie was always so positive about these things.

I had wanted to go to St. Thomas's Hospital in London to train for nursing. It was well-known as being *the* place for nursing training. But Mum and Dad would not hear of it, as it was too far away, and I think they felt that London was a den of iniquity.

So I applied instead to Bristol Royal Hospitals for a place on their training programme, which consisted of practical time on the wards with lectures interspersed for several months every year for three years, by which time, assuming I passed all the examinations, I would be a State Registered Nurse: SRN. Mum came with me to the interview and answered all Matron's questions for me. Matron looked rather surprised, but I was accepted with no problem, as my educational standard was satisfactory. I was still too young to start, so I went back to the sixth form until the end of the year.

At school, those who had passed the final examination were presented with the appropriate certificate. To my surprise, my school certificate showed my two distinctions, six credits and one pass (which was the way in which our marks were classified) and stated that my work had been 'very satisfactory'. I was amazed and gratified. At least I had something to *show* Mum and Dad this time, unlike the scholarship!

While in the sixth form, those who had chosen nursing as their future were assigned to the local college for three days a week to attend a 'pre-nursing course'. This did not carry any qualifications but was just an introduction to nursing. It was purely theoretical, dealing with the anatomy and physiology of the human body, an understanding of sepsis and its causes, the difference between a virus and a bacterium, some of the minor procedures that we might meet and the names of some pieces of equipment like spatula, swab, kidney dish, a mysterious solution called eusol and some dressings, with a brief idea of how these things were used. We were taught how to sterilise utensils, treat pressure sores, address patients and so on. All this was purely theoretical and taught in the classroom. It proved to be of minimal use once we were on the wards, as the ward sisters were gods of their own domain, and everything had to be done their way.

The lectures that I enjoyed the most involved the diagnosis of conditions by signs and symptoms and their treatment. Perhaps I *should* have been a doctor after all.

Eventually, I reached seventeen and a half, the age at which I could be accepted at the hospital, so, at the end of the term, my last day at school dawned. Once more, I stood outside the head-mistress's study. Miss Prestige had retired about two years ago, and Miss Banks had been appointed. She was not the gentle, lady-like person that the popular Miss Prestige had been, but a large, sarcastic woman with a grating voice. I went in when the green light showed, and, in a dismissive way, I was briefly wished good luck in my chosen career. Miss Banks seemed to disapprove of any career that did not involve maths, but I did not have the courage to tell her that I *would be using maths* to work out drug dosages. She would not have been interested, I'm sure.

So my school days ended.

Perhaps Bristol would be all right, I thought. At least I would be able to see the four-year-old Robert quite often as he grew.

No Longer 'The Child'

An ordinary morning in early September marked the last day of my childhood. I was no longer 'the child'.

My case was packed.

Everything that I owned was to go with me, it seemed. I did not have much anyway: a few clothes, some school notebooks, a sewing box and a few books. It appeared that, from now on, Meadow View would not be classed as my home and nothing of mine was to remain there. The nurses' hostel would be my home instead.

I waved to Mum and Robert and Tig from the car window as Dad drove me towards the rest of my life.

Into the Big, Wide World of Work

The Nurses' Home

Dad was quiet as he drove me towards Bristol and the next phase of my life. I wondered idly if he would miss me.

He was still very busy. The war had been over for four years now, and several of his workmen had returned from the fighting. They were all trying to get the Works back to its previously neat and tidy appearance, but Dad also had to ensure that there was a greater capacity for the treatment of waste water to meet the demand from an unexpected population increase. When people mentioned the boost in the birth rate, they spoke darkly of the presence in Bath during the latter part of the war of hundreds of attractive American GIs and the gullible girls who fell for their charms and their money, only to be left with 'illegitimate' babies when these young men went home.

We also still had Admiralty personnel stationed in some of the hotels in Bath. Foreign workers, too, seemed to have popped up from nowhere (actually from the erstwhile occupied countries) to help in the rebuilding of the shattered city; many people who had been bombed out were returning to their repaired homes or to the hastily constructed prefabs, so people were flooding into the area.

All these factors meant that Dad and his men were almost as busy as they had been during the war itself, when fire-watching and Home Guard duties had been added to the daily workload of the few who were not called up.

We drove into the outskirts of Bristol, another city ravaged by sustained bombing. Everywhere you looked, there were reminders of that terrible time: huge swathes of open ground where houses or offices had once stood and the shored-up ends of rows of terraced houses; rebuilding was in progress, and children were playing among piles of rubble and the remains of buildings. As in Bath, many such sites were softened by buddleia bushes and foxgloves, which seemed to flourish in any disturbed soil or piles of broken concrete.

I did not know Bristol at all, having returned only once since Dad had taken me away from the stucco bungalow, and that was for my initial interview at the hospital. I had been far too nervous then to notice anything of my surroundings.

'Where do we have to go, exactly?' asked Dad, as we approached the huge bulk of the hospital building.

'I think we have to go straight to the nurses' home in Tyrell Street,' I replied, naming a very steep, narrow side street.

We found the address and drew up before a green door over which were the initials of the hospital: B. R. I.

'I'll just drop you off here,' said Dad. 'I'm blocking the road.'

He put my belongings on the pavement, and, with a wave and a call of 'good luck', he was off.

At that moment, the door opened and a group of girls came out, laughing and chatting. When they saw me, one said, 'Oh. A new girl. Watch out for the Dragon!' And with these less-than-reassuring words, they ran off to catch up with the others, who roared at some joke.

I looked at the closing door. Should I ring or just open it and go in? At that moment it started to rain, so I pushed my belongings in through the doorway and followed, shutting it behind me. With the closing of that door, with Dad and the world I knew on the outside and me there alone on the inside, I felt it was the ending of something and the beginning of another: but the beginning of what?

Working—yes.

Freedom from home—yes.

But it was also something more. Perhaps at last I might be someone in my own right. I would certainly not be just 'the child'.

New Acquaintances

I was standing in a bare hallway with two staircases leading up from one side. On my right was a window with the word 'Reception' over it. A large woman with bleached hair, wearing a green overall, peered at me.

'Name?' she barked.

I approached. 'Brown,' I said.

'Two Browns. Which are you?'

'Julia'

'Ah. You will be in room 23 with Nurse Webster and Nurse Cleeve.'

'Are they new, too?' I asked.

'Of course. Only the new nurses have to share. Up those stairs—third floor, along the corridor, turn left, fourth room on the right. Here is a list of house rules. Any misdemeanour will be reported to the Matron.'

'Thank you,' I said. 'What do I have to do when I have unpacked?'

'If you want to eat, go to the dining room.' And with that she closed the window and returned to her knitting. Was this the Dragon?

The Country Nurse Remembers

It felt like the first day at a new school. Where was all this freedom about which I had dreamed? I pushed the list of rules between my teeth, as I needed both hands to carry my case, coat, sewing box and a small cardboard box of school books. At least I would know what the rules *were* here, and, to someone who had been subject to many incomprehensible rules, that at least was a comfort. I struggled up the stairs, along the corridor and eventually found room 23.

I knocked (it was instinctive) and waited.

The door was flung open by a hefty, rather forbidding young woman.

'You Brown?' I was to learn that Nurse Webster did not waste time on unnecessary words.

'Yes, that's me,' I replied, teeth still clamped around the rules, trying a nonchalant approach to cover my apprehension.

'In,' she instructed, holding the door open. 'First name?'

'Julia.'

'Oh, very posh.'

'Well, not really. Just my name.' I could see that I was going to have to be very careful with . . . It occurred to me I didn't know her name.

'What is your name?'

'Natalie,' she replied.

The door opened again, and a small, thin girl entered. She stopped when she saw me.

'Oh, hello. I'm Anna Cleeve. You must be Brown.'

'Yes. Julia.' This seemed better.

Anna smiled and pointed to the third bed. 'That one will be yours. I had to have the one by the window. My asthma, you know.'

I didn't know, of course, but I would learn that asthma was only one of a dozen or so illnesses from which Anna was sure she suffered. I began to put my clothes into the small chest beside my bed. There was only one wardrobe, so I hesitated before opening it.

'Not much room,' said Natalie. 'Not mine. All Anna's.'

I took my few things out of the old case.

'Gosh! That all you've got? Bad as me. 'Spect you left a lot at home. That right?'

'Oh, yes. That's right.' I was doing it again. Pretending. They might think that my parents were mean if I told them that this was all I had.

Why was I sticking up for home and parents again? I don't know, even now.

Conversation was stilted and intermittent. Although they had met some hours earlier, I think we were *all* wary of one another and *I* was afraid that I would not fit in. I seemed to know nothing about the things they were discussing. Anna knew the names of all the doctors and where the wards were and what to choose (when there *was* a choice) in the dining room, while Natalie had firm views on the type of training that she hoped we would get and voiced her intention of asking to be put on a surgical ward right away. Anna tried to tell her that we would go where we were sent, but Natalie would have none of it.

I looked at my 'rules' and saw that it was supper time.

'Is it all right if I go and have supper?' I asked

They gaped at me.

'Of course. Why not? We are coming, too.'

'Where do we have to sit?' I asked, as we collected our food from the counter.

Again, they looked at me as though I had two heads. 'Anywhere you like, of course,' they answered in unison. I saw Natalie shake her head, and Anna seemed highly amused.

I began to see that within the rules there was a freedom that was understood by the others. Although they were new, like me,

The Country Nurse Remembers

I was less at ease in this new environment. Natalie and Anna must have thought me very odd at the time.

We sat at the end of a long table where a number of second-year student nurses were eating and chatting. None of the snippets that we could hear were about work, and I would learn that you left your work at the door, so to speak, unless something out of the ordinary had happened.

A Senior Sister came into the dining room and clapped her hands.

'Sister Tutor,' hissed Anna.

Sister Tutor peered round. 'Are there any new nurses here?'

There was a chorus of 'Yes, Sister.' I glanced around and was delighted to see a familiar face—Margaret from my school was there, and I smiled across. She made signs that we should meet after supper.

Sister Tutor was speaking. 'All first-year nurses are to see me in the hall at eight p.m. for uniforms, and you will be allocated your wards for tomorrow.' And out she swept.

Anna and Natalie led the way to the hall. How did they know where it was? Out of politeness, I sat beside them but kept looking for Margaret.

Sister Tutor and two Senior Nurses, who were carrying piles of uniforms, walked onto the little platform.

'Good evening, Nurses.' Sister was addressing about fifteen of us, but I felt proud to be called 'Nurse' for the first time. She went on to allocate wards and shifts for the following day, and then the nurses handed out the uniforms. We had been measured at the interview and were now given about six plain white dresses, a maroon cape, a mauve belt and round pieces of starched linen.

'You will now watch Nurse Trendier as she shows you how to construct your caps.'

We learnt how to bend, button and form the caps, were told to be on the ward by 6:30 a.m. and then she bid us goodnight. Off went Sister and the Senior Nurses.

'What do we do now?' I asked Natalie.

'Take this lot to the room,' she said, as though addressing an infant.

'I mean after that,' I persisted.

'Whatever you like, of course, so long as you are in by eleven p.m.'

'You mean we can go out, if we like?' It was already 8:45 p.m.

Natalie looked hard at me. 'You don't know anything, do you?'

What she said only confirmed what I was beginning to realise. I still had so much to learn about being considered an adult, about making decisions for myself—even little ones. This was something that I had rarely been allowed to do. Other girls about my age seemed so capable, so confident and worldly-wise.

I shrugged, assuming a nonchalance that I did not feel. 'I just thought it was a bit late and we have to be up early.'

'Oh, she'll wake us, don't worry.'

'Who will wake us?' As soon as I had asked, I felt foolish. Here was something *else* that they knew and I didn't.

'Mrs. Smith. *The Dragon.*'

'Right.' I wanted to know if the woman at reception was the Dragon, but I didn't dare ask any *more* questions and seem even more of an idiot.

Just at the right moment, Margaret appeared. 'Found you,' she said. 'Let's have a natter.'

We found the sitting room, a large, sparsely furnished room. We sat and swapped impressions, and I found that, although she seemed much more confident than I felt, she too was a bit lost in the new environment. She came from a happy home in Bath and had not been away from her parents before.

The Country Nurse Remembers

'I miss home already,' she laughed. 'I don't know anyone except you. I wish we were in the same room.'

I did not miss home (but I didn't tell her that), but I too wished we were 'bunked' together.

'Do you think we could ask to be changed?' I queried.

'Doubt it. That would mean other people having to change.'

We chatted on. At school, we had been in the same year but not the same class and we did not have the same circle of friends, but here we were, both glad to find a familiar face, and we formed a friendship that evening that has lasted (albeit at a distance later in our lives) into the present.

I made my way to my bed and was asleep in no time, probably exhausted by all the new impressions or perhaps because it was eleven o'clock and I was not used to staying up so late.

The First Working Day

'Five-thirty, nurses!' the Dragon shouted into the room. Then—bang!—the door slammed shut.

I woke with a start.

The echo of 'Five-thirty, Nurses' passed on down the corridor, getting quieter as the distance increased.

I was out of bed like a flash, into my dressing gown and off to the bathroom while the other two were mumbling and yawning.

'You're keen,' said Natalie on my return.

'Well, we have to get up and have breakfast and then be on the ward by 6:30, don't we?'

'You bothering with breakfast?'

I looked at Natalie in disbelief. 'Are you not?'

'Nah. Have mine at coffee break.'

Passing up the chance of a meal was madness, I thought.

Anna said, 'I can't eat breakfast. My hiatus hernia, you know.'

Breakfast was quite substantial, if hurried, and then all who were on duty made their way across the gardens to a back entrance to the hospital. Now I knew why we were issued with capes: it was cold and wet running across those gardens.

Just inside the door stood a Senior Sister. Each nurse who passed gave her name, and it was ticked off on a sheet.

The Country Nurse Remembers

Woe betide anyone who had not left enough time to get to her ward by 6:30 a.m!

I made my way to the medical cardiac ward, which was a male ward, made up of two rooms each with fifteeen beds. It was right at the top of the building, with a panoramic view of the town—bomb damage included. I would learn that there was no time to look out of the windows anyway.

I reported to Sister Verne, a bustling woman with quick movements whose starched apron crackled as she walked . . .

'Yes, yes. Nurse Brown. Morning bedpans have been done, so you will be making beds with Nurse Tripp, and then you will do lockers and wash the bed patients. You might get backs done before coffee time.'

All this left me in a complete panic. I had hardly heard it all: my mind was trying to catch up with the last instruction as the rest were being fired at me.

'Brown!'

I turned. I had never been called by my surname before. Behind me was a smart third-year nurse who was looking at me.

'Let's get started. Have you ever made a bed before?'

'Only my own,' I replied, being unconsciously literal.

She laughed, thinking that I was purposely making a joke.

'Well, you won't have done hospital corners, then.'

What were hospital corners?

I soon found that there was a special way to strip an empty bed (if the patient had gone to the toilet, perhaps) and a different way for an occupied one; that each pillow was replaced with the open end away from the door, and that hospital corners were a very neat way of tucking the bottom sheet in; that a turn-over of the top sheet had to be exactly eighteen inches and that the other end at the foot was turned back by the same amount.

I had been silent throughout, but then I asked, 'Why do we turn the top sheet back at the foot?' It looked uncomfortable to me.

'So that we can turn it around at the evening bed-making if the top has got messy.'

Many patients, who were not too ill, read newspapers to pass the time, and the newsprint blackened the sheets (newsprint in the post-war years was very unstable). There were strict rules about clean sheets. If a long-stay patient had spilled anything or perhaps a wound had leaked, or there had been an 'accident', a clean sheet was allowed; but generally clean linen was doled out to one side of the ward one day and the other the next. Usefully, I learnt how to help a patient 'up the bed' while he hauled on the overhead handle, which was on the end of a rope hanging from the bent metal hoist, which was nothing at all like the hydraulic hoists in hospitals today. If the patient was not capable of this, the two of us had to move him about by holding him in the approved way. Some patients could be eighteen or twenty stone (252 or 280 pounds), and we were expected to manage. It was apparently possible, 'if you do it properly', we were told. This attitude led to many slipped discs and strained muscles in the nurses of the day. Luckily for us, there were no large patients in at that time.

'Doing lockers' involved removing any rubbish from the locker top, removing the water glass and jug and wiping the top with some foul-smelling antiseptic solution.

What had not been mentioned (and so far I was only doing exactly as I was told—there was no time for extras) was that doing lockers also involved taking the jugs and glasses to the ward kitchen, washing them, filling the jugs and returning them to the ward.

'Nurse Brown!' Sister appeared in the kitchen doorway. 'You have not laid up the trolley for washing the patients yet.'

'I'm sorry, Sister,' I apologised automatically. 'What do I . . . ?' But she had gone.

What on earth did 'lay up a trolley for washing the patients' mean?

Nurse Tripp came in to help me with the jugs and enlightened me. For almost everything, a trolley or tray had to be 'laid up' in the approved fashion. The 'patient washing' trolley had to have bowls, jugs of hot water, soap, flannels, towels, tooth mugs on the top shelf and a bucket for soiled linen on the bottom. Patients were kept in bed for much longer then than nowadays, so there were plenty of 'bed patients' to wash.

'Aren't you coming to coffee?' Nurse Tripp appeared in the sluice doorway.

'Is it time? I haven't finished all the washes yet.' I was staggered to hear that it was 9:30 a.m.—time for the half-hour break. It was a lot less than a half-hour by the time we had run down the four flights of stairs (nurses were not allowed to use the lifts), run across the gardens and climbed to the nurses' home dining room. There was scarcely time to gulp a cup of watery coffee and rush back *up* all those stairs. I wondered if it was worth it, but we were expected to do this marathon: it was in *the rules*.

Back on the ward, Sister bore down upon me.

'Right, Nurse Brown, you must look at the duty list in the kitchen in future, but because you are new, you will work mornings and afternoons this week. You have one hour for lunch and then you are back here until six. You then have the evening off.'

She made it sound like a gift to an undeserving child.

'You are very slow,' she continued, 'but l will overlook it, as you are new. It is time for the morning round, so be sure that the beds are tidy and the "up" patients are in their beds and don't have books or papers all over them. After the round, do the bed-pan round before the patients' lunch.' Then off she went.

There seemed to be endless 'rounds', but I supposed this one must be the doctors' round. It sounded very important, and once more Nurse Tripp and I rushed around the beds, whisking newspapers out of sight, tucking patients in and smoothing the covers. As the lowest of the low, I was told to get on with my work quietly while the doctors were there, but I was not told what I had to do, quietly or otherwise, so I skulked in the sluice doorway and watched.

Sister and Staff Nurse stood by the ward door, Staff Nurse holding a pile of patient notes. In came a very large, elegantly dressed doctor in an immaculate white coat, followed by two other doctors, not quite so tidy, and four student doctors who looked a little down-at-heel compared with the august presence of Professor Proud—as the eminent man proved to be called. Most appropriate, I thought.

Sister approached and accompanied the Professor and his entourage, with Staff Nurse beside her, handing her the patient notes at exactly the right moment. The Professor addressed the doctors and student doctors, imparting information and asking questions. They were obviously terrified of him. I sympathised, as I felt the same fear of Sisters and Senior Nurses.

The parade around the ward went well until one very elderly man shouted out, 'Nurse! Nurse, I be wantin' a bottle.'

Everyone ignored him. I did not know what to do. I only just knew what he meant.

Sister glanced towards him. 'Mr. Turner, can you please wait until the round has finished.'

I doubt if the old fellow knew what 'a round' was.

'No, that I can't. I be goin' to wet the bloody bed.'

I felt that, as the lowest of the low, bedpans and bottles were my responsibility, so I grabbed a bottle (and they looked like bottles then—they were made of glass) and quickly shoved it under the bedclothes. As I turned my back (as though he cared about that), I caught Sister's look of absolute horror and Staff Nurse's red, embarrassed face.

A much-relieved old man drew the almost full bottle from beneath the clothes and, in full view, handed it to me, saying, 'See, Nurse. I did want un' like I said.'

I scuttled off to the sluice, knowing that somehow I had done something very wrong and would soon be 'on the carpet'—but what?

The round ended and they all packed into Sister's office for a few moments, and I could hear the Professor holding forth. Then Sister stomped into the sluice, where I was trying to be invisible.

'What do you think you were doing, Nurse Brown? How dare you shame the staff and the patients in front of the Professor? I was mortified, and I have a good mind to report you to Matron.'

Oh no! Not on my very first day! What would Mum say if she got to hear of it?

I was literally trembling. 'I . . . I'm sorry, Sister, He wanted a bottle . . . I . . . I just thought I was doing the right thing.'

'The right thing? *If*—and it is an *if*—the patient really needed a urinal, we do not call that receptacle a "bottle" here, Nurse. You should have put two screens quietly round his bed and fetched the urinal covered by a cloth, and removed it in the same quiet way, taken it to the sluice and returned to remove the screens. There was no need for chat.'

I hadn't opened my mouth; the patient had uttered one sentence. I sensed that explanation would be unwelcome, however.

'I'm sorry, Sister.' I muttered, close to tears. 'I . . . I didn't know.'

'Hmm. I suppose not. It was most unfortunate. *Most* unfortunate! Well, I will not report you this time, but just be sure you do things properly in future.'

I was so relieved.

Some of the Patients

The next morning, Natalie got up in time for breakfast.

'I thought you had yours at coffee?' I said.

'Nah,' Natalie growled. 'They had cleared it all away by then. Miserable lot!'

'Well, I suppose they have their rules, just as we do,' I offered.

Anna, too, was making signs of getting up. 'I shall have to force something down, I suppose. Yesterday I felt quite faint by coffee time.'

Natalie and I had quickly learnt to ignore Anna's aches and pains—they seemed to change daily anyway.

On the ward, I started to do the same things as the day before and got through my duties a lot faster. I also made an effort to get to know the patients a bit, though standing talking was not allowed. If a nurse happened to have nothing to do for a minute or two (and this rarely happened), she would hide in the sluice because if Sister saw her doing nothing, even for a second, she was in trouble and judged to be lazy. The odd moment could have been well spent talking to some of the vulnerable or lonely patients; so this rule was most inconsiderate. It was also counter-productive, as sometimes nurses were deemed unfriendly.

The Country Nurse Remembers

One patient on the cardiac ward was a very caring man called Mr. Code (pronounced 'Codey'). Although he had ankylosing spondilitis, a severe type of arthritis affecting the spine, and was bent almost double, he pottered about the ward doing little things for the bed-bound patients, such as pouring them a glass of water from the jug that they could not reach or taking a letter to the ward post box, which was just outside the door. He was on the cardiac ward because he also had a heart condition that was being assessed. He had been in a long time, knew all the staff and wandered at will into Sister's office or the kitchen with little jokes or snatches of ditties. He would sing, as he pottered around, 'If I Knew You Were Coming, I'd've Baked a Cake'.

I was working in new surroundings with unfamiliar people, the terms of my work were still vaguely unknown and I was so dizzyingly rushed in all that I had to do that the fact that I remember him so well must mean that he was really exceptional. I have a warm feeling, even after some sixty-odd years later, when I remember him.

Heart disease in the 1950s was often fatal, as it was not well understood; drugs were only just being devised to treat the different conditions, and heart surgery was in its infancy. I remember young men who had collapsed at work, and older men who were unable to walk more than a few paces without having to pause for breath; some of the patients were blue about the lips because there was not enough oxygen getting through, and many days I would come on duty to find yet another empty bed.

In my first week, we admitted a double amputee. This man had been in a car accident and had had to have both legs amputated, one below the knee and one above. He was transferred from the surgical ward about a week after his operation to the medical cardiac ward because it was discovered that he had a serious heart condition. He was very ill and confused, and the screens were round him all the time. As the most junior nurse, I had nothing to do with him—he needed special care and was 'specialled' at all times by a Senior Nurse.

On my second day, however, the special nurse had to leave him for just a moment to fetch a clean gown, as he had vomited. As she rushed out from behind the screens, leaving them open so that other staff could see him, she glanced at me and called, 'Watch him for a second and shout if you need help.'

I was passing with some clean sheets. I put them on the end of his bed and stood looking at him. He was quiet and appeared to be asleep, but then quite suddenly he sat up and began to rip the bandages off one amputation. I shouted for help, but no one came. I tried to tell him to stop, but he did not understand; he did not even seem to realise that he had no legs because he began to get out of bed. Shouting again, I barely caught him as he fell to the ground, just as the nurse rushed back.

'Oh, no. Not again!' She helped me to lift him, or perhaps I helped her, and we got him back on the bed. He had opened the wound by pulling at the bandages, and the raw, weeping, bleeding area was exposed. It was the first time that I had seen an amputation wound, and, although quite shocked, I was glad to find that I was not revolted or disgusted. This was good. I desperately wanted to be a good, sensible nurse, so I thought this was probably a good test.

The special nurse called Sister, and they dealt with the dressings, for I was much too junior to know how.

'Psst! What's happened, Nurse,' a young man in the next bed whispered.

'Well, I . . . '

Sister overheard and cut off anything I might have said. 'Nurse, you do not discuss one patient with another.'

'No, Sister.' I answered. I had not been about to tell the young man anything other than that the man was 'rather poorly', but arguing with Sister, even to defend myself, was not a good idea. At least, I thought, I had been brought up never to argue, no matter what the reason, so humility came easily.

The young man said later: 'Nurse, did I get you into trouble?'

'No, it's all right.' There I was, pretending again!

'I wouldn't want to get you into trouble. I think you are so pretty. They make you work so hard—I think they are jealous.'

I had no idea how to deal with this: nothing of this nature had happened to me before, so I just smiled, shook my head and got on with my interrupted work.

Young Mr. Arnold (we were not allowed to use forenames) kept looking at me and trying to catch my eye. I was afraid Sister would notice. I felt gauche and inadequate; I was sure that all the other girls would have known what to say.

The day passed, as many were to do, in something of a blur of beds and bedpans, lockers and washings, feedings and turnings, taking patients to the lavatories, then more beds.

That evening I went to bed at eight p.m. I was too tired even to chat with Margaret.

A First

The man with the amputations, whom I will call Mr. Jones, was very ill and not expected to live for many more days. I heard it said that there was nothing else that could be done for him except to ensure that he was comfortable, which meant sedated. I thought it strange and sad to think that we were there (as doctors and nurses) to make folk better, but we were just waiting for a man to die. This was something that I would get used to in time, as various terminally ill patients came and went, but the first time it felt like a corporate failure. I wished that I could talk to someone about my confused feelings, but the ethos of that ward at least was that we just got on with whatever we were doing, only asked essential questions and obeyed orders and did not voice 'feelings'.

Feelings were not allowed; it was not done to exhibit them. I wonder if this strict rule accounted for the stern looks on the faces of so many Sisters and the fact that consultants on their rounds rarely spoke *to* their patients: only about them. After the many years that some Sisters had been following this rule, their sympathetic side must have shrivelled. I did not have time to think all this out then, but I have wondered about it since. Times are very different now; in many ways, we have become too informal and unprofessional, even sentimental, and perhaps hypocritical.

Late in the afternoon on one of my first few days in the ward I was told to take something to the nurse who was looking after Mr. Jones. As I opened the screens, he gave a deep gurgle and died—just like that. One minute, his eyes were open and he was breathing; the next, there was this strange sound and he was dead. I just stood holding whatever it was that I had in my hands, slowly realising that I was looking at a dead person for the first time. I must have looked shocked because the nurse gently took the thing from me and quietly pushed me out through the screens.

I knew about death—oh yes, I knew about death! My mother's death had changed my childhood (in fact, my whole life), and all the deaths in the war had depleted families that I knew, taking friends' fathers and brothers. But so far I had been spared the sight of a dead person.

I carried on with my work, but when my break came I could not join the others in the dining room as usual. I needed a little time to come to terms with my feelings. We could not entirely suppress them, after all.

A Day Off

Just as I was going off duty at six p.m., or just after, Sister called me. What had I done wrong this time, I wondered, as I made my way to the office?

'Nurse Brown, have you looked at the days-off rota and the duty hours for next week?'

'No, Sister, not yet.'

'You should look at the list every Monday morning before you start your work.'

'Yes, Sister. Thank you.'

I was to have a day off on Thursday, so, with Margaret, who was luckily off at the same time, I made plans to wander around Bristol, looking at the shops. We were thinking about going to a restaurant for a coffee but decided to have one in the dining room instead. Not so nice—but free!

I rang home from the call box in the hallway. The Dragon always managed to be around when anyone was phoning and listened to the end of any of our conversations. It was thus not possible to tell anyone what we really thought of the Sisters and doctors, as she would report any criticism to Matron.

Mum answered, and after the usual hellos I told her that I had Thursday off.

'Oh, good,' she said. 'That will be useful because you can look after Robert. I have a hair appointment, and I was wondering how I'd manage.'

'Oh, but Margaret and I were going to have a look around Bristol.' As soon as I said it I realised it was wrong!

'What? I'm not having you wandering aimlessly round town. Just come home and look after your brother.'

So that was that.

Odd that Meadow View was still my home when I was needed there. I found it very difficult to tell Margaret and managed to make it sound important that I should have to look after Robert. But my heart sank. Was I going to have to go home for every day off? I loved young Robert and was already making plans to save some of my forthcoming (and meagre) salary to buy him a toy car, but I had hoped to have some days off to myself. Freedom seemed to be fading. Perhaps I was a fool to think that it would be easy to begin a life of my own.

Robert was pleased to see me, and Dad was mildly interested in my work but seemed strangely bothered to know that I was working on a men's ward. Who did he think nursed the men? Mum found me useful, as I dusted and polished—it was as if I had never left.

As I left to catch the bus back to the nurses' home, Mum called after me: 'See you next week!'

It was obvious that I would have to do any wandering round town in my mornings or afternoons off.

The nurses' rota divided the day into three periods: mornings (6:30 a.m.–12:30 p.m.), afternoons (12:30–6:00 p.m.), and evenings (6:00–9:00 p.m.). Night duty began at 8:30 p.m. (so that there was an overlap) through until six a.m. There was half an hour for coffee or tea and one hour for lunch. We had either mornings, afternoons or evenings off, but if we had the morning off, we still worked from 6:30 to 9:30 a.m., and then we were free until 12:30 p.m. (with lunch at noon). Evenings off were the favourite: off at six p.m. and we could have supper or not as we wished, and most nurses went out to dances or pictures, perhaps with a boyfriend, and we felt like the rest of the working world.

But we had to be in by eleven p.m. We were allowed a late pass once a week. The Dragon was always there at eleven p.m., looking pointedly at the minute hand on the huge clock on the wall. If we had a late pass, she was there staring at the same minute hand, pointing usually to a few seconds past one. So when did she sleep?

Night duty was quite different. Six nights on and two off for three months at a time. During this spell, it was very difficult to pursue any social life, as we were going to work while the rest of the world was going out for the evening. Our nights off were often spent catching up on sleep. We lost touch with our friends, especially any boyfriends, who just seemed to fade away in the face of our non-availability for dates.

The night nurse's home was on the Downs in a quiet street, but although we were on nights, the cleaners worked in the day, so there were vacuums whirring and buckets clattering about. I hated night duty with a passion! I found sleeping in the day almost impossible, so I was always tired.

I became friendly with a Welsh girl called Joan, and we began to get to know the centre of Bristol, still only partially rebuilt, but of interest to two country girls. Young women of today would wonder that we found anything in the shops to interest us, but the wartime shortages had been such that any clothes or shoes *now* on display were exciting. For the first month of my training (before we were paid), I had only enough money for the bus fare home and back for my days off, so I could only *look*, but my ambition was to buy a pair of high-heeled court shoes—the height of sophistication at the time—

followed by the car that I wanted to get for Robert. I knew that we would only be paid £5, so I should have to budget. The car would cost £4 and would leave me once more with only £1 for the rest of that month. But I was sure that Robert's delighted little face would be well worth it!

Moving On

I worked on the cardiac ward for about three months. I admired Sister but was terrified of her: she was so quick at everything, including her speech. She had a Welsh accent and spoke so very fast that I had a great deal of trouble following instructions—I was still trying to work out what the first one was by the time the next two or three had been fired at me. I remember one day when I was testing urine for sugar (a newly acquired skill), Sister rushed into the sluice.

'Nurse . . . h . . . you see . . . a lum . . . punt . . . ?'

That is how it sounded to me. I thought something was lost and she was asking me if I had seen it, so I just said, 'No, Sister.'

A while later, she came in again and this time spoke in disapproving tones. 'Do you mean that you would be *ill* if you watched a lumbar puncture?'

I said, 'Oh no, Sister. I wouldn't.' This was the sort of thing that I was interested in. (It would also make a worthwhile change from urine testing.)

She looked surprised and a little puzzled. 'You mean you *would* like to see one?'

'Oh, yes please.'

The Country Nurse Remembers

Sister continued to look at me for a moment, gave a small sigh and motioned me to follow her. Why did I not tell her that initially I had just not understood her? As it was, she probably thought I was rather odd.

I made another terrible gaff without knowing it. The doctors' round was being done, so Sister and Staff Nurse were both in attendance when the ward phone rang. At first I ignored it, as juniors were not supposed to answer the phone in case they gave out the wrong information. But no one else appeared, and it continued to ring.

Staff Nurse looked away from the doctors and motioned to me to go and answer it.

With trepidation, I picked up the receiver.

'This is Doctor . . . ' I didn't catch the name. 'I wish to speak to Dr. Stern. It is urgent.'

'Oh . . . yes,' I muttered and hurried into the ward where the junior doctors were listening to the consultant, Dr. Stern, with rapt attention. I approached the great man and coughed slightly to gain his attention. He gazed at me with his eyebrows up, and I quietly gave him the message. He hurried away, and I looked around. Sister and Staff Nurse wore thunderous expressions, while the student doctors gazed at me with a sort of amazed respect.

Oh, boy! What had I done now?

'My office, Nurse,' said Sister in menacing tones.

She stood behind her desk. 'Do not ever, *ever* do that again. Who do you think you are, addressing a consultant like that.'

'I'm sorry, Sister. I thought I was polite, and the message was urgent.'

'You are only a junior nurse. You have been on the ward for no time at all, and yet you think you can address a consultant *yourself*. Only the Ward Sister or, in her absence, the Staff Nurse in charge addresses consultants. Have you learnt nothing in your time here?'

I was beginning to understand at last. 'I'm sorry, Sister. I did not know that rule.'

'I am ashamed of you . . . Such inappropriate behaviour . . . A disgrace!' She ranted on, and it was only the return of Dr. Stern that made her stop. Then she was full of charm and propelled him off to the ward again.

My colleagues seemed to know of this rule when I told my tale of woe. Why had I not heard about it? I seriously began to wonder if I might be deaf.

I was due to move on to a surgical ward the following day, so I collected my record, which detailed my progress on the cardiac ward. I was certain that it would be awful and silently thanked the Good Lord that Mum need not know. I took it in to supper unopened.

'Aren't you going to open it?' The other juniors, who were also moving on, were astonished. On the whole their records had been quite good, although Anna's remarked that it was the patients who were supposed to be ill, not the nurses. A reference, no doubt, to her constant stories of this or that complaint that she imagined she had.

'No,' I said. 'I know it will be bad. She'll say that I am slow and rude and don't listen and so on. I hardly need to open it.'

Margaret snatched the envelope from me and ripped it open. She handed me the sheet of paper.

I unfolded it with trepidation. 'Wow! Oh my!'

To my amazement, the record was quite good. I was a hard worker, neat and tidy, good with the patients, was learning quickly but needed to listen to instructions more carefully. Perhaps I *was* deaf because I always listened carefully but still seemed to get some things wrong.

The Surgical Ward

If the cardiac ward had been my baptism, the surgical ward was total immersion. Again a male ward, it was housed in one enormous room. There were fifteen beds down each side and an 'overflow' ten down the middle. These had little privacy, as there was no wall behind them and hardly any space between them to arrange the cumbersome screens which we put around beds to attend patient needs. The ward was only supposed to have thirty beds at most, but these were the post-war years, and hospitals all over the country were still dealing with people who had been on the waiting list for surgery for much of the war, while emergencies from the bombings, returning military personnel and those suffering as a result of wartime privations were dealt with. Now they were trying to catch up, so the extra beds, originally erected for the wartime casualties, were left in order that ordinary folk got their long-awaited surgery. I was amazed at how understanding most people were, in spite of having been in pain for perhaps years.

The distances we had to cover in such a huge ward were punishing, and we (the new young nurses) found that the only way to ease aching feet was to place books under the legs of our beds at night, thus raising the foot end by ten or twelve inches. I don't know who first thought of this, but it was a blessing, enabling us to reduce the throbbing, and sometimes swelling, of feet and ankles. I suppose our legs and feet eventually got used to it because I do not remember raising my bed for more than a few weeks, partly because the down side of this system was that during sleep we gradually slid downwards and found our heads pressed painfully against the iron rails of the bed-head.

I loved that ward! In spite of the speed at which everything had to be done, the air of hope was stimulating. It was a general surgery ward, so hernias, stomach ulcers, various lumps and bumps (usually benign) and internal investigations were dealt with routinely, while emergencies such as appendicitis were whisked in and to theatre between the 'list' patients. The surgeons and theatre staff worked very hard to reduce the backlog, but it took a few more years, partly because new and more complicated surgery was being introduced all the time.

I was now getting faster at the things I knew and learning all the time. I could take blood pressure and deal with sterilisers—there were no disposable needles or syringes, and the metal and glass reusable ones had to be boiled in a shallow, rectangular saucepan on the stove in the ward kitchen. This was time consuming and often resulted in broken syringes. When the needles had been used and boiled a number of times, they formed a barb on the end. If we used them without noticing, the patient would very soon tell us. But giving injections was still a long way ahead for me.

There were some larger, electrical sterilisers for kidney dishes, round bowls and instruments for doing dressings. There was also a fearsome washer affair for the metal bedpans and glass urinals. This thing rattled and hissed and blew steam everywhere but was loved by all the nursing staff, as it had only recently been introduced. Before that, we had had to wash the bedpans by hand!

The early mornings whirled by in a blur, rushing to get patients due for an 'op' that day 'prepped'. This meant washing, shaving the operation area, preparing the bed in a certain way and urging the patient into a theatre gown. The shaving was the worst part.

The area to be operated on was usually the abdomen, which involved shaving a very intimate area of a man's body. If there was a male nurse on the ward, he did the shaving, but there were few male nurses then.

At this particular time, the male nurse allocated to our ward was starting the following week, so it fell to me to do the shaving. As a new, very young nurse, I found this most embarrassing. The young men tried to laugh it off with various doubtful comments, while the older ones felt deep embarrassment—and often resented the indignity. I think the Sisters and other experienced nurses could have handled the matter better, rather than throwing us in at the deep end. I, for one, had no idea that handling a young man's intimate parts could cause unintentional excitement and embarrassment for him, and total confusion for me. I did not have the social skill to cope with this and turned my back the first time it happened. I waited a while and then carried on, but my action probably made him think that I was disgusted or disapproving. There was a tension between that patient and me for the rest of his stay.

The episode left me in shock; as well as being awkward I had no idea of the 'mechanics' of the male erection. Obviously I knew about intercourse, but I did not know that what was happening was usually a necessary part of it all.

As men from the RAMC (Royal Army Medical Corp) were demobbed, more male nurses or orderlies were recruited by the hospitals, so the female nurses were spared this minefield of embarrassment.

Natalie was completely at ease with shaving, and some of my colleagues were inclined to giggle. Anna was predictably 'ill': 'I have such bad nerves, you know. I find these young men so crude—it makes me quite ill.' Perhaps they had not experienced the same reaction I'd seen, of a man's excitement. They didn't say and I couldn't ask.

When the porters came for the ops, a nurse had to go with the patient as far as the anaesthetic room. I was most intrigued to see all the equipment on the anaesthetic trolley and to be among the white-robed figures who hurried about their tasks with such quiet confidence. Would I ever aspire to be so organised, so knowledgeable?

'The Bloods'

The surgical wards always seemed to be full of young doctors (housemen) and medical students. The more senior of these students were there to assess patients before operation—their findings were checked by the doctors—and to take blood for cross-matching in case a blood transfusion became necessary. Inevitably, they were known as 'the bloods'.

One of the more senior nurses, Clarissa, seemed to have caught the eye of one of the bloods, who made valiant attempts to talk to her. He had to choose a moment when she was working at the far end of the ward or when Sister was occupied elsewhere. This kept proving impossible, as either a doctor would call him or Sister would appear at the wrong moment. In the end the resourceful man slipped a note to a cooperative patient, who then waited for Clarrisa to pass his bed.

'Psst!' he said as she passed.

She did not hear. He repeated his call more loudly: '*Psst!*'

Clarrisa still did not hear, or did not think the summons was for her.

But Sister heard.

'What is the matter, Mr. Turner? You are sneezing a lot. Have you a cold? If so, you should have informed the hospital when they sent for you. We do not want cold germs here.'

'No, I am all right, Sister. Really I am.' He looked accusingly at the blood. 'I don't want my operation to be put off.'

'Hmm,' said Sister. 'I shall be watching you, and if you sneeze again, we will have to send you home.'

'I won't, Sister. I won't.'

I saw all this from the other side of the ward. The blood's face was puce, as the patient scowled horribly at him. He snatched the note back, then marched down the length of the ward so that he would pass Clarrisa, who was still blissfully unaware of the drama. Without a word, he stuffed the note onto the tray that she was carrying, turned and walked out. A very startled Clarrisa must have replied because they went out together and eventually, after he had qualified and she had passed her finals, married and lived in blissful poverty.

She became one of the very few married nurses that we had. A married girl was not allowed to train and take the nursing exams. One or two married during training and kept it a secret, as they would have been dismissed instantly, even if they were near their finals. Once qualified, however, a married woman could work, but on a part-time basis only. I have never understood these unfair, wasteful and pointless rules.

Many of us thought that the bloods were handsome and impressive in their short white coats (the doctors wore long ones). In comparison, we were usually too busy or too lowly to be noticed.

Sveto

Onto the ward came a slight young man with a beard. He disappeared into Sister's office and emerged wearing a white short-sleeved tunic. Sister clapped her hands for anyone nearby to pay attention.

'This is Sveto Pannitskeya. Sveto is a doctor in his own country of Poland, but our training is different so he cannot practise as a doctor here, but he can be employed as a nurse. It was difficult to place him, as he is the first such person to come to the hospital, but Matron has put him at the stage of a third-year nurse in training. He will need to get to know our ways, and you will all be of help where possible.'

Sveto smiled and said thank you in very good English but with a pronounced accent.

Sister turned to me. 'As he needs to understand the system from the bottom up, I suggest he works with you for a few days.'

I was pleased and worried at the same time. I had never had anything to do with foreigners apart from the German prisoners of war, and Dad had not allowed me to even talk to them. Sveto was just called 'Sveto' because his surname was so difficult. He did all the menial tasks with me, but when we started to take the patients' blood pressures and pulses, he was so much faster than

I was that we zipped around quickly. Bed-making, however, was a closed book to him; he kept saying, 'Why?' about hospital corners and turning over eighteen inches of sheet. I had not thought how odd and unnecessary it all must seem to someone who was not brainwashed, as we were, into thinking that it was the *only* way to do these things.

Obviously, he could not be accommodated in the nurses' home, so he slept at the YMCA, which he praised highly. At the end of a day spent with him, I knew no more about him than at the start, although I guessed that the reason for his presence in the UK was likely to be sad.

After supper, he thanked me for 'looking after' him, then said, 'I expect you will be wondering why I am here in your country?'

I think he wanted to talk about his circumstances, but stupidly I said, 'Oh, it's all right.' This could have sounded discouraging, but luckily he did not take it that way.

He told me about his family in Poland before the war: his mother, who was from a Jewish background, and his father, who was a surgeon. The Nazis arrested his mother and sent her to a concentration camp and tried to press his father into doing experimental operations on Jewish people. I discovered that my horrors were still with me from the time that I had seen the newsreel about the German atrocities. As he spoke, I found that I was sweating and my heart was beating very fast; I didn't want him to go on because I was afraid of what I might hear. Luckily, my inability to speak about those things prevented me from being foolish enough or unkind enough to stop him.

His father refused to cooperate with the Germans and was shot. His mother also died in the camp. Sveto did not know if she had been killed or tortured or starved. As I listened, I realised that I was talking with someone who had been close to the horrors that I had only seen on the newsreel and I felt ashamed, but even so I wanted him to stop—not tell me any more about his mother and the camp.

I was also ashamed for another reason: Sveto could not stop the tears, as he remembered his parents and their terrible end. I had never seen a man cry. My father was a tough Lancashire man; the rest of the male members of his family were much the same, and in that culture men did not cry. As my nursing career progressed, I would see many a man cry, either from pain or at the death of a dear one, but so far that had not happened and Sveto's tears embarrassed me. I knew that they shouldn't, but I had to look away from him. I don't think he noticed.

'What about you?' I asked eventually.

He smiled sadly. 'I had just passed my finals, my sister was a nurse and we knew that with the Jewish connection and our useful skills we would be either used for the same kind of work that they had wanted Father to do—and we agreed that we could not do that—or we would be killed off as being of no use. We left our home one dark night, creeping from shadow to shadow until we were out in the countryside. We were trying to get to Sweden, which was neutral, but it was wintertime and we were often cold and hungry. We tried to get food and shelter at farms along the way, but many people were too frightened of the Nazis to help us.

'After months of walking, sometimes begging and sometimes even stealing food, we were about a day away from the sea. We hoped to persuade a fishing boat to take us out into the Baltic and perhaps transfer us onto a Swedish boat, but the port was patrolled by Nazi troops.

'We were slinking along a road in the dark when we heard a shout. It was a German trooper raising the alarm. We had already decided that if this sort of thing happened, we would not give ourselves up—we knew what our fate would be—so we ran. Elise was shot in the back, I in the shoulder. I knew she was dead, so I kept going and somehow I escaped. I was numb with misery after her death, but I kept going. I *did* get on a fishing boat, and I *did* get transferred to a Swedish boat. I was befriended by a fisherman's wife, who hid me from just about everyone. You never knew if someone was a German sympathiser, you see, even there. I worked at whatever I could and after the war I came here, but I was very ill with TB. So I have been in hospital for three years. I am cured and fit now, so I need to work.'

After a moment, I said, 'What are you going to do? Can you go home?'

He shook his head. 'The Russians would come after me. You see, I killed a man. A Russian. He lived in Poland before the war, and he had raped Elise. I knew where he lived, and while I was on the run from the Germans I found him and . . . I killed him.'

I didn't know what to say. How do you react to someone who tells you that he has killed a man? He glanced at me and must have seen the confusion in my face.

'No, it wasn't in cold blood, as that sounds. I was going to give him a beating. I had a heavy stick. But I was weakened by starvation and illness, and I was getting the worst of the fight. He had me pinned to the ground in the barn where I had found him and was trying to strangle me when I felt something beside me. It was metal and heavy. With what strength I had left, I hit the back of his head as he bent over me. He died instantly.'

Sveto gave a huge sigh, which seemed to come from the depths of his soul.

'So you see, I have to stay here where I am safe until I can think how to prove that I killed in self-defence. I didn't want him dead. I just wanted to give him a beating for Elise.'

He stopped talking and sighed again, as he rose to go.

'I should not have bothered you with all this, but it is a relief to talk to someone sympathetic.'

The Country Nurse Remembers

I was glad that he thought so, but if he had known my real reactions and reservations, my horrors and my wanting him to stop, he would not have felt that he had a sympathetic listener at all.

'See you tomorrow,' he said. 'What shift are we on?'

He left, nodding to the other nurses. I suddenly realised that we must have been the subject of much scrutiny and gossip, as we were sitting at a separate table.

Natalie came over. 'You have made a hit there,' she said.

'No, it's not that at all. He just wanted to talk.'

'Oh, yes?' She did not believe me, but I could not tell her what we had really been talking about, and I realised that there would be gossip. I hoped that Sveto would not hear it!

The Toy Car

It had taken me longer than I had anticipated to save up for Robert's toy car, as I had had to buy another pair of 'duty shoes'. These had to be brown lace-ups with a rubber sole. My original pair had been black; they had been tolerated because I was new and I had explained that they were the only suitable shoes that I had. After a month or so, the Sister who seemed to be in charge of the nurses' welfare lost patience and ordered me to get the correct uniform shoes. They were known as 'Oxfords' and were good shoes but expensive for the time—about £2—while ordinary shoes could be bought for a little as a pound. This had cut into my previous month's salary of £5.

My day off was coming up, so I went to the toy shop and excitedly bought a pedal jeep with full camouflage paint. I staggered back to the nurses' home with it to the vast amusement of the Dragon as I passed through the hall. She found equal amusement the following day when I departed for my day off complete with toy car. The bus conductor was more understanding.

'I'll put un in yer,' said he, as he stowed the car under the stairs of the double-decker bus. I sat where I could keep an eye on my precious purchase and proudly carried it the considerable distance from the bus stop to home. Robert came to the door, as he had seen me coming up the road. I had tried to keep the car behind my back, but he could see that I had *something*.

I put it down on the front path. Robert ran to it and immediately jumped into it, his grin as wide as his face.

'Is this for me?' he asked.

'Of course it is!' I could see how thrilled he was.

Mum stood in the door with a look of amazement. 'Where did you get that?' she asked.

Taking her literally, I answered with the name of the toy shop.

'You mean you bought it?'

How else did she think I had acquired it?, I wondered. 'Yes, of course. I've been saving for this, but I had to buy shoes last month or he would have had it sooner.'

Mum was silent. Meanwhile Robert was 'vroom-vrooming' his way down the path. I dumped my belongings on the step— wow, I was getting brave!—and ran after him.

Mum and Dad had moved from Meadow View, and in front of the house they now lived in there was a circular path around a grassy area, so Robert and I spent some time going round and round on the path, but he was not good at steering yet, so there were many spills and lots of laughter.

Dad was amazed when he came home.

'I thought nurses were badly paid,' he said.

'They are,' said Mum, to my surprise. 'But she saved up for this car for Robert.'

'It must have taken nearly all your money,' observed Dad.

I was now confident enough to laugh, as I said, 'Yes. Nearly.' I didn't know how, but I felt that a barrier of some sort had been overcome and that I was talking to them as an adult.

The 'adult' thing did not last. But Robert's joy was what mattered, and that was very apparent.

Dancing

Sveto and I worked together for several days, as I showed him the job of a new first-year nurse. One day he said, 'What do you do when you have an evening off?'

'Not a great deal,' I replied. 'I haven't much money. But when I can afford it, I go to the pictures with friends.'

'Do you not go dancing? Young ladies in my home country love to dance.'

'I do, too,' I said. 'Sometimes the university has dances and then I go with other nurses, and the medical students usually ask us to dance.'

'Ah, I see. Well, I belong to a very nice dancing group,' Sveto explained. 'We go to dances in the big hotel ballrooms.'

'That would cost far more than any of us could possibly afford. How on earth do you afford it?'

'I have some money. After the war, the Polish authorities got in touch with me and gave me my father's compensation money and what little my parents had in the bank. So I am not, as you say here, "broke".'

I blushed as, belatedly, I realised that I had been rude to ask. I was used to the other nurses always talking about how they couldn't afford this or that, and it hadn't occurred to me that

Sveto might be different. I should have been more discreet because he was twenty-six; he wasn't just a young person straight out of school like the rest of us.

'Would you come with me?' Sveto asked.

'Sorry?'

'I asked if you would come with me—to dance. Or do you have a boyfriend who would be jealous?'

'No,' I said. 'I mean no, I haven't a boyfriend, and I would love to go dancing with you.'

'Good. The ladies usually wear long dresses,' responded Sveto.

I think he guessed that I would not own such a thing and was warning me. I thought rapidly: 'I could borrow one.'

Sveto smiled, and two evenings later we went to a smart hotel, one of the few that had escaped the bombs and still clung to its pre-war opulence. People were well dressed, except many of the men were only in lounge suits while the women were in evening dresses. I had borrowed a rather childish white dress with puff sleeves, but it was full length. I promised myself that I would get something better as soon as possible.

I found that Sveto was a very good dancer—at last my dancing lessons were useful. With such a good 'lead', I could do all the moves, and we danced together very well.

'I have to be in by eleven,' I told him.

'Next time you must get a late pass,' he said, obviously intending us to go dancing again. I was delighted, as I loved dancing and I liked Sveto, although he seemed remote. Polite and correct—but remote. I could not tell what he thought about the dancing or me, and he never did refer to his past again. It seemed that having once made me aware of his circumstances he just wanted to concentrate on the present. Or perhaps he was just waiting to be able to return to his own country and his career as a doctor.

We went dancing whenever we had evenings off together. I bought a beautiful pink evening dress for a few shillings from a girl who was leaving to get married. I had that dress for years. It had huge dark-pink flowers on it and was well cut, with an accentuated waist and low neckline. I loved that dress!

I was silly enough to tell Mum and Dad about the dancing. Mum had liked dancing when young, and I thought she might be interested. Wrong! Mum did not like the idea of the pink evening dress, and Dad was horrified that I had 'taken up' with a foreigner.

'I don't think you should have anything to do with this man. You have to remember that the foreigner is not like us.' He was very stern.

I was wise enough not to argue or ask in what way 'the foreigner' was not 'like us'. I was told not to see him again outside the hospital. I managed not to actually promise, but I think they were under the impression that I would do as I was told.

As it happened, I did not see him again, in or out of the hospital. When I returned from my day off, Sveto was not there. He was now working with a second-year nurse to learn the skills expected at that stage of training, but he should have been in the hospital. I overheard the second-year nurse say that the Ward Sister had expected him. Why was he not around, then?

I asked the nurse.

She seemed quite concerned. 'None of us know why he has not turned up for duty. He was always most punctual and a very good worker, and Sister is making enquiries at the YMCA, where he sleeps.'

But the YMCA could not shed any light on his disappearance: he was paid up to date, and his belongings, such as they were, had gone. I liked Sveto and I wondered worriedly if this had anything to do with the man he had killed, but I obviously could not mention this.

The Country Nurse Remembers

It would be nice to be able to say that he turned up with some good reason for his absence, but that did not happen. We never saw him again, and, to this day, I have no idea what happened. It was as if he had never existed.

At least I was able to tell Mum and Dad that I was no longer seeing him.

I missed the dancing. As I look back, I wonder how any of us had the energy for such things. But I heard that a military camp a few miles distant was putting on a dance for young officers and had sent an invitation to the nurses' home. It was a fairly frequent event apparently, as many of the men were away from home and had little money to spare for amusements. Rather like the nurses!

The camp sent a minibus for us, and those lucky enough to have the evening off dressed in our evening dresses, if we had them, or best short dresses if not, and set off for an evening of dancing, light supper and fun!

'Fun' was very necessary, as we dealt with sickness and death all the time.

We had all obtained late passes until 1 am and the bus driver knew that he had to get us back by that time, but when we assembled at the camp gates, there was no sign of him or his bus. The guards were not too helpful, so we stood about wondering what to do.

A very smart, older officer came by, and we told him our tale of woe. He immediately ordered one of the guards to investigate. We waited and were eventually told that the minibus had broken down out in the countryside while on another job. The officer immediately ordered a staff car and driver, and all seven of us squashed into the big Humber. No seat belts then!

Inevitably, we were late. It was 1:30 a.m. when the car dropped us outside the hospital. The nurses' home was in darkness (the Dragon must have gone off duty), so we had to go through the hospital entrance. A Deputy Matron sitting at a desk just inside looked at us and pointedly at her watch. We explained what had happened and showed our late passes.

'Hmm. I understand that it was not your fault, so I shall not need to send you to Matron. I shall ring the camp in the morning to complain. A group of young girls should not have been left waiting with no explanation.'

Whilst relieved that we had got off lightly, we were very afraid that if the Deputy made a complaint we might not get asked again. We staggered off to bed for a meagre four hours' sleep, and for the first time I was very glad that the Dragon had such a loud voice when calling: 'Five-thirty, nurse.'

Learning All the Time

The three-month college time began. I was delighted to be learning so much, not only about nursing procedures, but also about the human body, the diagnosis and preferred treatment of various diseases, complications to look for and the chances of complete recovery. Heart surgery was in its infancy and new drugs for heart disease were being discovered all the time, so there was great excitement in that field.

Much of the nurses' work we had already done on the wards, so this part seemed a waste of time to me, though I think our practical skills had overtaken the theoretical teaching because of the rush to try to catch up with the 'list' patients, many of whom were still awaiting operations or treatment four years after the end of the war. We still worked on the wards from 6:30 to 9:30 a.m., then departed for the college, where we spent the day until six p.m., with a break for lunch. College also meant that we had the evenings off.

Much of our time off-duty was spent in the nurses' home, chatting with friends and colleagues, because most of us had only our salary of £5 a month and so the pictures and dances were out of reach a lot of the time. I was delighted to have any money of my own at all and at first was almost surprised that my work was rewarded in this way. This sounds quite ridiculous now, as it probably did then to some, but I think my gratitude for pay was a result of having done a great deal of housework at home for no reward. I'm sure many other girls helped at home, but my work had been wrapped up in the myth that Mum was teaching me useful skills, when in fact scrubbing floors, dusting furniture, beating carpets, polishing lino and washing up were the only things I was taught, and I did those over and over for years and years, only learning anything new when Robert came along: then I added baby care to my accomplishments.

Other girls seemed to have learned a bit about the cost of things, or how to cook, or care for plants or clothes, but they were not expected to do the same thing all the time. When I was still at school, I used to listen to girls talking in a very grown-up fashion about how such and such was done or how you made a certain cake or why you washed and ironed some garments and dry cleaned others. Some even talked about the government or the council or, perhaps, what was going on in London or the recovering countries in Europe. I knew nothing of all this and had so far had no inclination to find out. I was still, in effect, a child—one who had always waited to be told things, had not thought for herself. It was just as well for me that the discipline and ethos of the nursing training at that time was so much like school—maybe boarding school. I would have been completely at sea if I had had to find my own accommodation, pay 'rates' or income tax or budget for heating, lighting and food; in fact, anything beyond trying to stretch next month's £5 to cover a new pair of shoes or a present for Robert or my bus fare 'home'. The first money I had handled was aged seventeen, when I was allowed the price of the dancing lessons. (Those wonderful dancing lessons that I was so glad I had had!)

The Country Nurse Remembers

So now to be taught practical skills on the wards—new things almost daily—and theoretical learning of such immense interest, and to actually be paid for doing it, seemed a small miracle.

One of my cousins had a holiday job while at university and was unhappy with his pay, which he felt should have risen when he was given more responsibility. He told me that he was going to ask for more. I was horrified that he should even think of asking for more money! Why, we nurses had to line up once a month, accept our pay packet and say, 'Thank you, Sister,' in a humble manner. Sister Ackerson accepted the gratitude as though she had personally reached into her own purse to pay us.

But apart from occasionally putting my foot in it through ignorance or misunderstanding, or perhaps carelessness, I was very happy in my training—on duty and off.

Fire and Water

There were still times when I made mistakes or was in trouble because I had not understood some instruction or perhaps had done something that was considered 'inappropriate'. One day was a complete disaster. In fact, two disasters, as one was the reason for the other.

I was in charge of the sterilisation of the syringes, of which there were many that morning. I arranged them, wrapped in gauze, in a row in the shallow saucepan, filled it with water and set it to boil on the gas stove in the ward kitchen, which was a little way along the corridor outside the ward itself.

Because of the next disaster, I forgot them. When I eventually remembered and rushed to the kitchen, I was greeted by smoke and a frightful smell. The pan had boiled dry, and about eight syringes and most of the needles were burned, as was the gauze surrounding them. The kitchen maid was happily drying some dishes and appeared not to have noticed. (She was a 'special case' employee; in other words, one who had special education needs but was quite capable of routine kitchen work.) Something out of the ordinary, it seemed, like smoke, was too much for her to comprehend.

I was in deep trouble with Sister, who told me that I would have to pay for new syringes. Luckily, when Matron heard about it and the reason why I had forgotten—which I shall explain shortly—she was cross with Sister rather than with me, which was most amazing.

'What nonsense!' she said, 'Of course you do not have to pay for the syringes.' And that was the end of it. But I don't think Sister liked me much after that.

The other disaster that day was the reason for the first.

We had two large, hard-working domestics who took their duties very seriously, deeming the nurses' work less important than theirs. We, the younger nurses, were terrified of them. They were always complaining that we were in their way, saying how did we expect them to do this or that if, for some reason, for example, we were late doing our duties (making the beds, for instance, because as we finished each bed we pulled it away from the wall so that they could sweep or vacuum behind it. They would stand and glower at us until we caught up.)

This particular morning, there were many bed baths to be done and only two of us to do them, so we assembled all that we would need for the several patients who we were attending at the end of the long ward and loaded up a trolley. On the top shelf of the trolley were two tall, steaming jugs of water.

We were pushing it very carefully down the ward when the front wheels caught in an uneven board in the floor, stopping its progress with a jerk. Both jugs fell forwards, spewing hot water all over the polished floor for about eight or nine feet, the spillage spreading as it went. We were rooted in horror and trepidation—not of Sister but of the domestics. Those two worthies stood by, huffing and puffing and not offering to help, as we spent some thirty minutes mopping up. We apologised and pointed out the uneven board, but they seemed to think that somehow we should have known about it. We said it had not been noticed before, how were we to know?

Luckily, Sister had seen what had happened and told the two grumblers, in no uncertain terms, to be quiet and find something else to do whilst they waited for us to finish. They went off muttering about having to polish it all over again and how 'these young nurses' didn't appreciate how hard they worked and so on.

That was when I remembered the syringes!

I don't imagine that we ever caught up with our schedule that day.

The Ball

The medical students held dances at the university from time to time, and I went to quite a few, usually by managing to change my off-duty times with accommodating friends. I could not understand why some of my colleagues did not want to go to these balls, as they were grandly called: Natalie was scathing, while Anna found them too noisy. I think, on reflection, that my dancing lessons were the reason I enjoyed such evenings. It meant that I was confident when students asked me to dance—I knew the steps and seemed to have a natural ability. Many of the students were not good dancers, but now and then a real dancer, with an appreciation of rhythm and a knowledge of the steps, came along. Then, when he discovered that I too could really dance, we might spend the rest of the evening together. Sometimes this would lead to being asked out, maybe to the pictures or some other dance-related event.

Contrary to a commonly held myth, *young* nurses and doctors very rarely went out together. To become a doctor took about six years, so most were in their mid- or late twenties, while we were still in our late teens. It was only the Staff Nurses and sometimes young Sisters who became romantically involved with doctors.

There was one notable exception, however.

Pearl was one of my first-year colleagues. She went to see the young doctor who was assigned to the nurses' sick bay that day because of a persistent cough. She sat in front of his desk, explained her problem, received a prescription and was just about to leave the room when he rose, strode to the door and held it open but in such a way that he barred her exit.

'Nurse Winter,' he said, 'will you have dinner with me?'

She was so taken aback that she could not speak for a moment.

'Tomorrow evening? I will pick you up at seven.'

'Yes. Thank you. I'll be ready.'

As a result of this, they went out a couple of times and eventually got engaged. Pearl did not even finish her training, as they married a few months later. Such a speedy and apparently seamless romance, however, was rare. Most students were on grants so, like the nurses, had no money for 'dinners'. A cup of coffee was about as romantic as it got for most of us.

A group of nurses of all stages in training were going to the university ball, and we all had late passes. The evening went well, and I got to know a bearded medical student because he was a fairly good and confident dancer. He talked almost non-stop about all manner of things. I was always glad if my partner talked a lot because I found myself very short of chit-chat.

I realised that I had little knowledge of anything outside the hospital, compared with many of the students; I still had not formed the habit of listening to the news or reading the newspapers, so I couldn't talk much about current events. Was this a hangover from my childhood years, when it was deemed wrong for me to do either? Or was it laziness on my part? In any case, we were rarely off duty at the right time to listen to the news on the one and only radio in the nurses' home. There was no television, of course—that came into general use several years later. Perhaps these are only excuses and I should have been more aware of the world around me.

The Country Nurse Remembers

I found that I was very innocent, too, in ways that perhaps a nurse should not be. I did not understand many of the jokes or stories that the patients and some of the nurses told, although they were not necessarily grubby, but just 'grown-up'. My father had always been against any suggestion of 'smuttiness', as he called it, and never told or tolerated doubtful jokes.

Martin, as the student was called, took me in to supper. We danced and talked, so I relaxed and we found a few things in common. At the end of the evening, he asked to take me home. It was a fine night, and I fondly thought we would walk through the quiet streets in the moonlight. I was even prepared to kiss him 'goodnight' in spite of the beard!

At the door, he said, 'I'll just go and get—' I did not hear the rest. A car, I thought, with respect. Very few students or nurses had cars.

But round the corner came a large, shiny motorbike. I was wearing a white evening dress (which I had bought from my friend and altered). I was going to have to ride pillion in a white evening dress! But I liked Martin and was not going to allow a little thing like my first-ever ride on a motorbike—even one in a white evening dress—to spoil a budding relationship.

So I bundled the folds of the skirt up around me and straddled the pillion, hanging on to Martin as though it were the most normal thing in the world to be whisked around at midnight in Bristol in an evening dress on a bike.

We went out together for some weeks and I had many rides on that bike, but I didn't tell Mum and Dad.

Night Duty

About halfway through my first year's training, my first spell of night duty loomed. I dreaded it. I had two days off and then would have to move to the night nurses' home. Here we had separate rooms in a big Victorian or Georgian house. Mine was on the first floor overlooking some neighbours' gardens. This was to prove a blessing a few weeks later.

My first night duty was on another forty-bedded surgical ward, this time housing women who were in for abdominal surgery, such as gastric and duodenal ulcers, appendectomies and the removal of the gallbladder, so it was a very busy ward for two nurses to run with only the help of an orderly.

The workload was heavy from the moment we entered. Last drinks to take round, last bedpans to do, the Senior Nurse had temperatures and blood pressures to take, and then the drug round. In spite of all this, we were expected to learn details about each patient from their names, ages and illnesses to the number of days after surgery, what drugs they required and at what intervals, whether they were allowed out of bed, if they were allowed food (and the same about drink in case of an operation the next day), any dressings, any special diet and sadly who, among the very ill, was likely to die. So often death came at night, when life is at its lowest ebb.

This sounds impossible, but I was lucky: I had the strange ability to rattle off all this information about all forty patients within the first hour or so. I have often wished that this odd ability extended into other parts of life—people's birthdays, shopping lists, recipes—but that flash of brilliance only worked on the wards.

I had a very pleasant and understanding Senior Nurse, so I learnt the routine quickly, and I soon realised why some nurses preferred night duty. You were almost your own mistress when in charge, because there were only two Night Sisters on duty and their visits to each ward were infrequent, except in the case of an emergency or some real difficulty. The Senior Nurse could apportion work and keep her own records, and so long as the jobs were done and her report to the Day Sister was complete, she could feel that she was 'boss'. If the nurse concerned was at all disorganised or even a bit sadistic, the junior could have a very poor time, so I was lucky.

Perhaps I might have liked night duty better had I been able to sleep in the daytime. Two or three hours' sleep seemed to be my limit, however, so I was always tired.

My new-found motorbiking friend, Martin, faded away as evening after evening he rang and I was not available to accompany him wherever his slightly mad ideas took him.

'The Window Incident'

I had returned from my days off at four p.m., as required, ready to have a couple of hours' sleep, if actually I managed to doze off. It was a bright, sunny day and my room was hot, having been closed up during my absence, so I decided to open the window. This had never been easy, as the windows were huge, almost floor-to-ceiling. They were double-width sash windows (the sort that have a rope running up a groove at the sides), with heavy wooden frames. I had to push the bottom window up as far as it would go in order to reach outside to grasp the bottom of the top window.

On this occasion, the window seemed to be stuck, and I had to get a better grip on it to pull harder. To do this, I put my hands between the two windows and pulled. There was a snapping sound, and the top window came hurtling down onto all my fingers, trapping them very painfully between the two heavy windows at about head height. In great pain and unable to move my hands or the window, I stood for a moment. I don't know what I was hoping for, but I did not want the indignity of having to yell for help.

Then of course, I had to.

I shouted many times over my shoulder, willing another nurse or the manager of the home to hear. But it was four in the afternoon: nurses would be asleep, and the manager's office was on the floor below. In desperation, I turned towards the open window. I could see some people in their gardens, so I shouted again and again.

Finally, I saw two men jump over their fence, rush across a garden and then there was a furious ringing at the nurses' home doorbell. A moment later, the manager, three men and a woman came into the room and began to heave at the window. There was a babble of voices while the men tried to push the window up to release my hands. They must have known that this would hurt me even more, but it was the only thing to be done. But the window defied them. One of them went off to get something, and two or three nurses arrived. Someone tried to take some of my weight because I had entered a state of shock and was almost hanging from my trapped hands, as my knees gave way.

At that stage, I think I moaned because I could hear *someone* moaning, but things were getting a bit hazy. Then I heard somebody say, 'It would be better if she *did* pass out!'

The efforts of these kind men were eventually rewarded, as they managed to push the window up enough to release me. Then I think they let go, and the window crashed to the floor. The nurses laid me on the bed, and I managed a rather weak 'thank you' to the men. The manager took me to the casualty department, and I received very prompt treatment. A young doctor had to drill into all my fingernails to release the blood which was gathering beneath them. Had he not done so, I would have gradually lost all my nails and been incapacitated for a long time. This was a very quick and simple procedure, but I smiled when this young doctor padded and dressed the finger ends and said, 'Keep the hands out of water.' I was a young probationer— did he not know that my hands were *always* in water?

I was allowed the night off, sleeping in the nurses' sick bay while they moved my possessions to another room until the window should be mended. In the next few weeks, I spent much time trying to work out the location of the houses viewed from that infamous window in order to leave a note of gratitude. I left several in possible doors—and at least one must have been right because, in addition to the telephone enquiries that the manager had received, one man added that it was 'not necessary' for me to thank him. 'We were put on this earth to help people,' he said. They were all such nice people.

The story grew in the telling, I think, because a local newspaper reporter came to the building and was promptly sent off by the manager, with the proverbial flea in his ear.

My fingernails were fine, in spite of constant immersion in water!

The young doctor would have been horrified.

Duck and Shout

I had been transferred to a men's ward part of the way through my night duty. This was unusual, and I do not remember why it happened, but this night there I sat at the desk, with the light on, preparing the treatment book for the following day. My senior colleague was at 'lunch' (midnight) and we had no orderly, so I was alone in a for-once quiet ward.

Among our patients, we had two men from the nearby psychiatric hospital. One was in for an appendectomy, the other for some urinary problem. As they needed close supervision, they were both located near the desk; they were inclined to shout a lot but had been sedated for the night. So peace reigned.

Suddenly, one of them roared for a bedpan (although he did not put it quite like that). I took one to him and slid it under his bottom. At that moment another patient called from the opposite end of the ward. Knowing that this long-stay patient would only call if it was important, I went to him immediately, leaving our friend on his bedpan. When I went back to retrieve it, however, the patient appeared to be asleep. Although I always think it must be most uncomfortable, patients frequently fell asleep with bedpans beneath them, especially if they had been sedated. Knowing his rather volatile temper, I left him and would remove that receptacle as soon as he stirred.

I returned to the desk to resume my task. It must have been a slight sound from his direction that made me look up—just in time to see a shiny metal object hurtling towards my head. I ducked! Indeed I ducked! I had no wish to be brained by a bedpan that might even be full. The pan travelled over the desk and landed with a terrible crash on the floor, spilling its contents: yes, it had been full.

I calmed the patient, who seemed to think that I had forgotten him and so had devised this somewhat extreme way of attracting my attention. Then I cleaned up the mess. The noise had woken half the ward, which, to a man, needed bottles or bedpans.

When my senior had departed for her meal, she had left a sleeping, peaceful ward. She returned to mayhem. It took us some time to settle everyone again.

But the 'fun' was not over yet.

The other patient from the psychiatric hospital had bed sides around him. These were rather like stalwart metal fencing attached to the bed frame so that the man could not climb out. He had a habit of removing every stitch of clothing, and, before he was constrained, he would make his way to the front entrance of the hospital, intent on escape. This had happened at visiting time, and legend had it that several elderly ladies had to be treated for shock. Whether this was true or not, we were taking no risks.

This man required four-hourly injections, which had to be done through the bars of the 'cot sides', as they were called. I happened to be longer in the arm than my more senior colleague, so, after she had drawn up the six am drug, I was going to do the injection. I talked to the man (we did not know if he understood us, but it was the practice to tell the patient what we were about to do) and reached inside the bars with my right hand, which held the syringe, and my left, to hold the man's leg steady. As I inserted the needle, the patient suddenly sat up and grabbed my arm.

The Country Nurse Remembers

The syringe went I know not where, as the man pushed my arm backwards against the bars, obviously intent on breaking it. I screamed for help. There were several healthy young men at the far end of the ward who were awaiting operations for such conditions as hernias, and three of these lanky fellows charged up the ward. Two of them held the patient—not too gently—while the third prised his hands from my arm. They looked thunderous: it was fairly unusual for a patient to attack a nurse, and they were furious that anyone should do so. I was bruised and sore but unharmed, and once more the centre of attention and concern.

Night Sister was called, but I convinced her that I was fine and told her how the young men, who were still standing by, as though to protect me from any further danger, had rushed to my aid. She smiled at them, thanking them but urging them back to bed, as they were in for operation that day. I was very grateful, too! They delighted in telling anyone who would listen how they had saved a nurse from injury. At least we did not have a reporter knocking on the door this time.

I cannot help but compare the way in which the incident was resolved with the fuss that there would be if a similar thing happened today. I am sure there would be meetings and forms and reports and investigations into procedure, staff safety would be scrutinised and maybe there would be pressure to make complaints and to sue someone—anyone who could be held responsible. We did make the psychiatric hospital aware of the incident so that extra vigilance could be maintained on his return. But that is all.

So my first spell of night duty drew to a close. It had not been short of excitement!

A Disappointment

I had a week's holiday straight after night duty. Mum and Dad had been thinking of taking a break themselves, and Dad was talking about going to see Auntie Jinny. Mum was not keen but seemed resigned.

When I arrived home on the first day of my holiday, I asked, 'When are we going to see Auntie Jinny?'

'What? Oh, we aren't,' said Mum. 'At least not for a while.'

I was deeply disappointed. 'Oh, that's a shame,' I said. 'Is it that Dad can't leave the Works or something?'

'Oh no. I just don't feel up to it. I get headaches in the car.' Mum had never had headaches in the car before.

'What does the doctor say?' I asked.

'Oh, I haven't bothered with the doctor.'

There was something else here, I thought, and wisely left the subject. But it meant that I spent the whole week at home, dusting, polishing, scrubbing. We visited Mum's parents in Bath—her mother was getting rather frail—and I wangled a visit to Grandma and Grandpa and Auntie Lizzy by myself but on my return was asked many questions about what they said and what I said and had they said anything about Mum and so on. There was definitely something odd going on, I thought.

The Country Nurse Remembers

At the end of a rather unsatisfactory week off, I returned to the nurses' home to find that I was to work on gynae for three months and then there would be another college session. Joan, the Welsh girl with whom I had become friendly, was assigned to the same ward. Things were looking up.

The next day there was a letter from Mum to say that they were going to visit Uncle Jake and family for two days, so I wouldn't be able to go home for my day off.

'Why can't you go home if you want to?' Joan asked.

'They won't be there,' I said, matter-of-factly.

'So?'

I looked at her for a moment and then realised what she meant. I was seventeen, nursing sick people, earning money, and I certainly knew how to behave in the home. Why was I not to go home, even if they were not there? It had never occurred to me, but I now saw that I had never stayed in the house without them. I had babysat Robert while they went out for the evening but had never been 'let loose' alone in the house for any other reason.

When I looked at the rest of her letter, I saw she had written: 'While we are at uncle's, we shall visit Auntie Jinny.' It was like a smack in the face! Why could Mum go to both Uncle Jake's home and Auntie Jinny's, when she could not go to see Auntie Jinny because of headaches in the car?

'Never mind,' said Joan. 'For some reason, they have given me the same day off, so why don't you come home with me?' Joan grinned as she said, 'Mum will be there.'

I knew that she was teasing.

So I went with her to the little cottage way out in the country not far from Raglan. We had to go by train, which went through the Severn Tunnel. This was a weird experience, especially when we stopped because of some hold-up on the line ahead. The silence was eerie and broken by the steady drip, drip of water from the walls and roof. This is apparently normal but is a little worrying when you remember that above you are hundreds of gallons of sea.

The cottage was tiny, with just the two bedrooms, so a mattress was put on the floor for me in Joan's room. There was no inside toilet or washing facilities. We had to go to a wash house in the garden, where there was plumbing and a huge boiler for hot water or to boil the linen. I loved the hot steamy atmosphere and smell of clean linen in that little place.

Joan's father worked on the railway and always left very early in the morning, so we only saw him in the evenings, when we would sit in front of the fire and tell stories or we would play board games. This was long before television. A lot of people had radiograms to play their records, but there was no sign of such a thing here. There *was* an old radio, but it didn't work anymore. In spite of the lack of such entertainment—or perhaps *because* of it—these were jolly, cosy days, with lots of chat. It was a little family of three people, each as important as the next. They lived and 'worked' as a unit. I was so impressed!

I spent many happy days off there and only lost contact with Joan years later when we were both married and living in different parts of the world.

When I told Mum where I had spent my day off, she seemed disapproving, but I don't know why. I asked after Aunt Jinny and was told that she was 'all right' but nothing more.

'Did she send me any message?'

'No. Why should she? You didn't send her one.'

'But Mum, I didn't know you were going until your letter . . . ,' I explained.

'You could have rung us.'

'I only got your letter when I came off duty—it was too late. You would have been on the way by then.'

'Oh, we didn't go when I said. We went the next day.'

The Country Nurse Remembers

I gave up and dropped the subject. There was no point in trying to have a proper conversation. Mum had made up her mind to be grumpy, it seemed.

There seemed to be an odd atmosphere on my next day off. I tried to ignore it, but something was wrong.

'I'll take Robert round the green with his car,' I said.

'Don't you mean, *May I take Robert round the green?*'

I looked at her and at Robert. I turned and went upstairs to the room that I stayed in when at home. The guest room—I had not had a room of my own since leaving for training.

What was happening? Things were worse than ever.

And was I not to be able to take Robert out to play when he or I wanted?

Church

Joan and I were wandering round the town, off duty, one afternoon.

'Let's go and look at the church,' she said. 'I have been in there before and it is beautiful.'

So went in to St. Mary Redcliffe. As we walked quietly round, we became aware that a service of some sort was in progress in a side chapel. We slipped in at the back, looking and listening in awe. The church was beautiful and grand—so unlike the church in my village. The service was littered with sung prayers, and bells were rung now and again. Finally, we realised that people were taking communion.

That day made us both think. We wanted to know more.

We had both been to church schools: I to Church of England, Joan to a Welsh Nonconformist school. At the first opportunity, we saw one of the clergy, who was very solemn and well-spoken, but welcoming in his restrained way. We made a date to see the Canon with a view to being confirmed.

We attended classes (not always together because of duty) and learnt the catechism, and answered questions about our reasons for wanting to be confirmed.

What were my real reasons? Not just that I liked the church, or the solemnity of the services, but that I had left behind my childhood association with the Christian faith when I left the village church school. The assembly services in the Grammar school had been brief and not inspiring, and I missed the simple faith that I had been taught in the junior school.

Mum professed herself to be a Methodist but rarely attended chapel. She had arranged for me to be christened, however, when she discovered from my father that this had not happened when I was a baby. I was nine at the time and I was now grateful to her, as I was able to tell the Canon that I was baptised. He was a rather splendid man—quite frightening, but he taught us well. We were confirmed by the bishop, together with about a dozen others, at a special service in this splendid church.

Mum was not too pleased that I had chosen Church of England as my faith rather than Methodism (Dad was an atheist—so he said, but I wonder if he really was just undecided), but Auntie Lizzy had a white dress made for me and bought me some pale grey shoes. The three of them and Joan's parents came to the service. The classes and arrangements had taken about a year, so the confirmation was held when we were both in our second year.

I wrote to tell Auntie Jinny about it all, and she was very pleased, saying that Mummy would have been pleased. I had never heard that my mother went to church very much, so I asked Auntie about this in my next letter. Her reply was typical of her unquestioning faith: 'Even if Mummy had not chosen Jesus, He had chosen her to be with Him because she had been a good and loving person.' She sent me a white prayer book with the date of my confirmation on the front. I treasured it for years and carried it as a bride.

I wish I could say that I followed the faith well and regularly, but I frequently 'fell by the wayside'. We had a lovely little chapel in the hospital, and I sometimes went to the Sunday service or just to be quiet if there had been a sad case, or if I felt that I had not dealt with something well, or if I was upset when things were not good at home.

Looking back, I think I must have had a rather frivolous side, so my faith was perhaps not always to the forefront of my life.

Swimming

The next college session was during a spell of superb weather. We finished lectures at six p.m., then about five or six of us rushed to the nurses' home for supper, gathered our swimming costumes and boarded a bus for Portishead, a small town on the Bristol Channel.

The sea around the Severn Estuary is brown and would be considered uninviting (and possibly polluted) now, but it was the nearest place accessible to us. And we loved it!

It would have been seven before we arrived, but, undeterred, we normally found a low rocky headland and stripped off. We had been there at low tide, so we were aware of the depth of water at high tide and spent the rest of the evening throwing ourselves into the murky water from a fairly high point. We dived, jumped, 'bombed', separately or hand in hand, for an hour and a half, then dried (a bit) and jumped on the last bus back to Bristol. I wonder now that we found it worthwhile, but oh we did!

Of course the times of high water were not always in our favour, but we had a little yellow book of tide times, and as soon as it seemed possible again, off we went.

I don't know when we fitted in the necessary 'swotting' for first-year exams, but, to my surprise, I did very well. Matron always took an interest in promising nurses and must have considered me to be worth her attention, as she sent for me to talk about my continuing training.

Matron was a round Scottish woman with a well-developed sense of duty to the hospital. Our uniform rules included keeping one's hair short or 'up'. Should a few locks stray below the permitted length, Matron would steam down a passageway, shouting, 'Keep your haaair off your collaaaar, nurrrrse,' and some frightened, tousled-headed nurse would scuttle to the nearest bathroom mirror to perform wonders with bobby pins.

On this day, I went before her mightily pleased with my results.

After a few preliminaries, Matron asked, 'And what do you like best about your nursing so far?'

I had already decided in what direction my future would lie. 'I like the college time and the lectures, Matron.'

Instead of being interested, she looked shocked. 'You should *never* enjoy lectures better than looking after patients, Nurse. This is a disgrace!'

I tried to tell her that I wanted to be a Sister Tutor—that was my ambition—and that was why I wanted to learn how to *teach* as well as how to nurse, but she had made up her mind that I was. . . what? Unfeeling? Lazy? I was dismissed without being able to defend myself. I was unhappy to be so misunderstood, but I had had good training in this at home.

Looking back, I think this was all part of my really wanting to be a doctor. But that was never going to happen.

Plans

I began to save up again. I wanted to go to see Auntie Jinny and it seemed that, for some reason, I was not going to be taken with Mum and Dad, so I set about finding out about train times and fares and the connecting bus. I had never done this before and found it rather confusing. The main problem was the cost. I could walk to the station in Bristol, catch a train to Cheltenham and then a bus to Winchcombe, but a return journey like this would take most of my month's salary and would take longer than my day off. I would have to ask Mum if I could miss spending my next week's holiday at home. I knew instinctively that she would not like it: there was something strange going on, to do with the non-visit before and my mother. How did I know all this? I had worked it out from snippets of conversation I had overheard between Mum and Dad.

It seemed that, for some reason, Auntie Jinny had written (she was no great letter writer) and had been unwise enough to mention that I had sent her a photo of me in uniform and how much I looked like my mother.

At about the same time, Mum had got it into her head that Dad was inclined to talk about my nursing rather than Robert's childish achievements. Dad had never been good at noticing things, but I was the first woman in the family to have a career, and he was quite proud of me. This came as a surprise to me, but, whilst I was glad, it was obviously causing trouble.

When I mentioned my plans to Mum, she said, 'Well, you can't go this next holiday because Grandma and Granddad are moving and I want you to help.'

I did not have any more holiday for a while but continued to save for the next one. I finally wrote to Auntie Jinny to say that I would be with her in two weeks' time. I did not hear from her, but a few days later there was my letter in the nurse's home box, returned to me.

I rang Mum and Dad. Mum answered, saying that the letter had probably just gone astray because of my bad writing. I didn't know what to do, so I wrote again—very carefully this time.

Goodbye

Auntie Jinny was dead.

What I felt was the last link with my mother had gone.

I was selfish enough to cry for myself, for the chats that we would never have, for the visit I would never make, for the assurances that I had been loved and so on.

After a while, I cried for the right reasons. That Auntie was no longer alive, going to her church, meeting her friends, living in her lovely cottage. That she just *wasn't* any more. She was no longer in the world.

Later still, I began to remember that she was sure that she would see 'dear Frank' when she died. Was she with him now? If so, I should be glad for her. But this was difficult.

Some friend of Auntie's, going through her address book, had written to Dad, and he, who never put pen to paper, had written to tell me.

I ended up going home at the beginning of the week that I had planned to go to Auntie's, but my parents were not there. I had no key, so I walked down through the village to see Grandma, Granddad and Auntie Lizzy. They told me that Auntie Jinny's friends had asked Dad to go and sort out her possessions, as she had no surviving relatives. That was where they were.

So after all that I spent my week off at the nurses' home. I went to Gloucester Road swimming baths, I wandered around Bristol, met up with some nursing friends and medical students and went to a pub for the first time. I went to church in the hope of gaining some comfort, but the place was in uproar and the services disrupted because there had been a scandal and one of the clergy had been 'defrocked'. Understanding nothing of the implications, we giggled about the term 'defrocked'; I went to the hospital chapel instead.

It was summertime and so there were no dances or balls, but a group of us took picnics onto the Downs and walked across the suspension bridge to the woods beyond. I went to the pictures twice because Laurence Olivier's *Hamlet* was being shown. My favourite actor and my favourite Shakespeare play all together! And, of course, I had some money to spend because I had been saving for the trip to Winchcombe that would never happen.

I said very little about Auntie Jinny because most of the girls would not have understood quite how much she had meant to me.

When I went home the following week, Mum seemed a bit less grumpy and showed me one or two plates that she had brought away from Auntie Jinny's cottage. Then she said, 'Auntie Jinny wanted you to have her sewing machine, but I knew you wouldn't want it, so we sold it.'

'I *would* have liked it, Mum.' Oh dear, I was arguing.

'What? Where do you think you were going to keep it? I don't want it here.'

So that was that.

I missed Auntie for a long, long time, but eventually I enjoyed remembering her and her cottage and all the lovely talks we had had about my mother and Jesus. As Mum and Dad rarely mentioned her, she became a kind of secret thought. If she was mentioned at all,

Mum's mouth took on the screwed-up position that she kept for people of whose opinions or lifestyle she didn't approve.

But without the bridge that Auntie provided between the times before my mother died and after, I was gradually finding it more painful to think about my mother and all the years that I felt I should have had with her. I didn't speak of her, either. Who was there now to hear me? My life was full of work, new experiences, new friends. I was forming opinions and had much to occupy me. I was growing away from the past and gradually building a future.

I don't remember exactly when it happened, but about then there was another sad event, when Tiggy had to be put to sleep. How I missed him! He had been so much a part of my childhood; so loved and cuddled, and the willing recipient of tearful confidences. His dark eyes and stubby tail said it all.

Better Times

I was now well into the second year of my training and therefore was given more responsibility and more interesting tasks to do such as administering different types of injections and other medication, putting on dressings, rehabilitation after operation, keeping of records and observation of the progress or otherwise of treatment.

Carrying out renal or rectal washouts were no one's favourite jobs, but they had to be done. Another procedure that I now did was 'Last Offices'—or 'laying out', to the layman. There was a very precise way of all aspects of this sad task. After washing and dressing the patient, you wrapped him in a crisp white sheet, which was pinned in place. Seven pins in all, facing the feet. This was most important! All this happened on the ward, no matter how busy we were, tending the living.

Today, all this is done in the mortuary or by the undertaker. But although it was time consuming and, perhaps, not the best thing to be doing among patients (albeit behind screens), at least the deceased was attended at his end by those who had known and nursed him.

Another night duty passed, thankfully with less drama than the first, and another college session was enjoyed—at least by me (in spite of Matron's disapproval)—and then I was assigned to theatre.

I was delighted, Bristol was at the forefront of budding technology and anaesthetics and was one of the very first hospitals to perform the famous, but now almost routine, 'blue baby' operation.

I was what was known as a 'runner'. We all started that way. We laid up the sterile trolleys with all the instruments for the 'scrub nurse' (more senior) to hand to the surgeon during the procedure. We learnt about sterile procedures and the correct order for everything, such as which masks and gloves had to be put on, and how to assist the surgeons and scrub nurse into their sterile gowns.

We had to learn the names of various bits of theatre equipment so that we could *run* for it when required. We cleared up after one op, washed everything down ready for the next and prepared the sterile drums of swabs and bandages. It was a very busy life, but I had the chance to watch various surgeons at work and observe the sort of thing that the scrub nurse did. How I aspired to be a scrub nurse!

`*

Much later, after I had finished my training and moved to London, I became a Theatre Staff Nurse for a time. The theatre was at the top of a very old building. One day, I was the scrub nurse assigned to assist an eminent brain surgeon, and we were operating on the brain of a seven-month-old baby who had encephalitis, which used to be known as 'water on the brain'. Gradually, we became aware of the blare of fire engines' sirens and the smell of smoke. I instructed my 'runner' to go to see what was going on. On his return (a male nurse this time) he told us that the fire was in the lower part of the hospital and ambulances were evacuating patients from all the wards.

The surgeon listened and carried on with the operation.

'We can't stop now. We will carry on for as long as possible. Any unnecessary staff can leave now,' he said, but no one did.

We all knew that the baby would die on the table if we stopped the surgery, so I ordered the fire doors to be closed and from time to time sent the runner to see how the fire was progressing. More and more fire engines and ambulances were arriving, but gradually the fire was brought under control, and at least some of the patients returned to their wards. The eight-hour operation continued as though nothing had happened. I was so very impressed with the selfless dedication of the team and the cool-headedness of the surgeon to be able to do this most tricky procedure on a tiny child with fire raging on the floors below. Such is the nature of theatre work that one only occasionally knows the eventual outcome of the surgery. The patient would be whisked off to a ward, would recover from the surgery and be discharged. Only very occasionally would we, the theatre nurses and technicians, happen to hear if he had lived or died. The surgeon would check up in the few hours after surgery and again at a follow-up appointment in Outpatients. The theatres were hectically busy, with no time for anything except the actual surgery and certainly none for following a patient's progress after operation.

It would be nice to say that the baby survived and lived on, but I do not know.

We found that every time we came back to the nurses' home from the night nurses' accommodation, we were given different rooms. Although I had been told that only new nurses had to share a room, there had been such an influx of new staff that we were still sharing into the second year.

Now, I was in a very large room with three other nurses; all second years. Not surprisingly, Anna had left. *This* made her ill, *that* gave her a rash, something else gave her nightmares and so on.

The Country Nurse Remembers

The final straw was when she was sure she had TB and Matron suggested that nursing was not the career for her. I do not remember where Natalie went, but she too seemed to disappear.

Margaret was in the next bed to me at the end of the room, and we had some good laughs and giggles. The other two girls were Plymouth Brethren. They prayed on their knees every night, they never listened to music, never swore (although the rest of us were pretty restrained), never wore make-up or talked about boys, only read the Bible or religious or nursing books and never seemed to go anywhere in off-duty time.

Della was tall and dark and very uncommunicative, but Cecilia (named after the patron saint of music) talked to us when she realised that we were interested in her faith. I don't think we understood why that faith was so repressive, but she was a good nurse and a gentle person and we respected her. But soon she amazed us all.

One day, the Dragon knocked on the door during the afternoon. Cecilia and I were off duty and reading.

'Someone to see you in the front 'all, Nurse Branden. A gent.'

Cecilia looked surprised. I was amazed. Normally, we were not supposed to have callers and certainly not 'gents'.

When she returned, she mentioned that it was her cousin, who had come to see if she would go out the following day. She had agreed to do so.

Our window overlooked Tyrell Street, so Margaret and I, being nosy, watched when Cecilia left the room. She was dressed sensibly with no high heels, no make-up and lisle stockings instead of the nylons for which the rest of us almost sold our souls (tights did not appear until the 1970s). There in the street was a red sports car, with a tall, handsome but far from stylish young man at the wheel.

In the following two or three weeks, Cecilia went out with him about four times: always in the daytime, always in the car and always returning completely composed.

'Nothing in it,' prophesied Margaret.

'No,' I agreed. 'She isn't the slightest bit excited.'

But we were wrong. The cousin, whom she had known from childhood but who had gone away for work, was now back with the extended Brethren family that ran a huge farming complex. He was 'courting' her in the old-fashioned way, having spoken to her father sometime previously to ask his permission to take her out and then to ask her to marry him.

The actual proposal happened in the bosom of the family on one of her days off, and she returned, still composed, wearing an engagement ring with a huge diamond in it. She put this away, and we only saw it if she was going out with the young man— most of us would have worn such a thing at every opportunity. . . though *not* on duty, of course.

One day, Margaret and I returned to the room to find Cecilia's bed neatly made, her chest of drawers empty and her case packed.

'I was just waiting to say goodbye,' she said. 'I am needed at home, so I shall not finish my training. I am to be married next Sunday.' She smiled at our amazed faces and was gone.

We later heard that his family had given them a house on the estate farm and her family had furnished it. They started a family immediately themselves and had six children in as many years.

Sick Nurses

I was on the ENT (Ear, Nose and Throat) ward for the second time, and for the second time I developed tonsillitis. I was placed at the end of the nurses' sick bay, far enough away from other nurse patients not to infect them. I received various treatments, which included a thick yellow penicillin intramuscular injection, which I now appreciated was just as painful as my patients said it was!

I recovered quickly on both occasions, but during my illness it was discovered that my sinuses were blocked. They were washed out (not a comfortable procedure), and suddenly the world became a noisier place; I could hear *exactly* what was being said *all* the time. So I *had* been a bit deaf, after all!

I was appalled to see three nurses with poliomyelitis at the opposite end of the room. Polio was rife in the early 1950s and was a constant hazard until the Salk vaccine was introduced in 1955. As a result of this and subsequent vaccines (such as the Sabin), polio is only found in India, Nigeria, Pakistan and Afghanistan today.

Nurses were particularly at risk because the organism is passed from person to person or is present in faecal matter. Before the introduction of automatic bedpan washers, nurses had to clean these receptacles by hand. With all the hand-washing in the world, there was still a considerable risk of contamination.

Two of the nurses were in the fever stage of polio: no one knew how much damage the virus had done and therefore how much paralysis would be caused. The third nurse was in an 'iron lung', as she was paralysed from the neck down. She could speak, see and hear, but the lung did the breathing for her. She was fed through a tube and given water the same way. A mirror was attached to the head end of the lung so that she could see what was going on around her. Cheerful and giggly, she was the star nurse patient of the era, but we all knew that her fragile body could not withstand for much longer the frequent infections to which she was prone. She died when I was in my third year. One of many sad cases at that time.

Ham Green

Out on a windy promontory overlooking the Severn Estuary near Avonmouth was a sprawling fevers and TB hospital called Ham Green. This sanitorium, or isolation hospital, was not really part of the Bristol Royal Hospital group, but it was in some way affiliated to it. Here were the patients with tuberculosis of the lungs, kidneys and other unusual locations, such as glands, and also those with rheumatic fever (or acute rheumatism), diphtheria, tropical diseases and polio. There was also a ward for smallpox sufferers. Situated by itself and fenced off, it was located some distance from all the others. While I was at Ham Green we did not have a case of smallpox, but it was not unknown for it to be brought in by returning troops or others from countries where that terrible disease was still rife. I was in the Middle East in the 1960s when smallpox raged through several nearby Arab villages almost yearly, killing countless people, mostly children. Widespread immunisation has now eradicated this terrible disease throughout the globe.

The other wards were also separated by large grassy areas with narrow tarmac paths, and there was a nurses' home, still with rules and regulations but at least there was no Dragon here.

When I went home for the first time after starting at Ham Green, I went to see Grandma, Granddad and Auntie Lizzy.

When I told Auntie that the wards were so far apart that many of the nurses and doctors used bicycles to get around, she immediately offered to buy me a bicycle. This was a lovely surprise, and the following week a Ladies Raleigh was waiting for me. The problem was that I had never ridden a bicycle and I had just a day and a half to learn!

I rode it back as far as the nurses' home in Tyrell Street, where I left it until my next day off, when I rode it the rest of the way. It made such a difference, not only getting to and from the wards, but also joining others on outings to nearby villages, including a little place called 'Pill'. Rather appropriate, I thought.

I was on the men's TB block. The treatment for TB was lengthy and the outcome uncertain in the days before antibiotics; it was based on rest, fresh air and a high-protein diet, and the patients were kept on bed rest for months. The TB block was made up of open-fronted cubicles. The head of the bed was against the back wall, and there were flimsy, movable walls on either side; the open front could be covered by a huge glass window, but this happened so rarely that most were rusty and unusable. In cold weather, the patients were tucked up beneath quantities of blankets, dressed in warm clothes and even gloves and woolly hats, and they looked out at the world of grass, trees, wind, rain and sometimes even snow. When it snowed, we covered the foot of the beds with a large, thick red waterproof rubber sheet and brushed the accumulated snow off from time to time. If this sounds amazing—it was! And we, the nurses, were still in our short-sleeved cotton dresses. It was surprising how many jumpers we could get underneath. But many patients owed their lives to such Draconian treatment.

In the case of children (and sadly there were many), the movable walls between the beds were rearranged so that two or more could be together. It seems incredible that so long as the patients were not too ill, they had *fun*. There was no tidy bed rule here, and models (complete with glue) were made; games, books, magazines and comics, colouring and sketching pencils and pads were in evidence daily. Even balls were allowed and were thrown to and fro, it being considered great fun if they managed to hit a nurse. They scored even higher if it was a Sister!

If the child was fit enough to have lessons, a teacher would gather some beds together (or rather we would), and a fairly relaxed and merry class would ensue. All staff, and that included the teacher, wore gowns and masks for any close contact treatment or prolonged exposure to the patients, which meant that in theory the teacher had to teach with a face mask on. Of course, it was only popped on when officials from the local Education Department came round. Everyone had been immunised against TB of course, but, even so, we ran ridiculous risks.

We had also been immunised against typhoid fever. This procedure involved two injections a week apart, the first being about half the strength of the second. Unfortunately, the young doctor assigned to this task happened to get the doses the wrong way round when I was due for mine. With a group of eleven other nurses, I was given the first dose, and, having been given the morning off, we all went into town. By midday, a fleet of ambulances had brought us back from all over Bristol—where many of us had collapsed or fainted. We all ended up in a row in makeshift beds in the sick bay. I felt about as ill as I ever remember feeling.

There was much consternation, and great minds at high level were consulted, but about twelve hours later we all began to feel part of the real world of our own accord.

The big problem then was what to do about the second injection: should the strength of this match the suggested first dose or should it be a repeat of the second? Whichever was chosen, I do not remember feeling so ill, so I think they must have given the lesser one.

We all had enormously swollen and painful arms, and it was all we could do not to screech when a patient, trying to sit up, caught hold at the spot.

The demographics in Ham Green were so different. Apart from the children, there were many young men who had been prisoners of war in Japan. Due to the deprivation, ill treatment, poor diet and lack of medical care, many of them had contracted TB, and many had had it for a long time. They would have been treated initially in military establishments, but this was now 1951 and the war had been over for nearly six years, so the men we nursed were those who had contracted the disease near the end or even after the end of hostilities, perhaps from undiagnosed friends. With only a few exceptions, those on our block were just about cured, were feeling fitter than they had for years and were almost ready to go home. They were mostly in their late twenties, young enough to need fun and willing to egg one another on. Young nurses were much admired but also badly teased.

It became known that I couldn't cope with spiders. The hospital was in the country, and the spiders were large and plentiful. Usually, I managed to avoid those patients who were known for their practical jokes and would sometimes chase me down the corridor with a large, hairy wriggling spider, but one day a devious fellow pretended to have a pain in his leg. As I bent over him, with my head positioned away from my collar, I felt the tell-tale tickle down my back. I can feel the clenching of stomach muscles even now as I remember the incident. And on that occasion I actually screamed—and fainted!

It must have been for a second only, as I heard several patients gasping, 'Oh my God!' Then I felt hands down my back, scrabbling about. There was a 'You've got it!' and an 'Is she all right?' followed more clearly as I came round by profuse and worried apologies, with much babbling about not knowing that people were *really* like this—not just pretending.

The Country Nurse Remembers

Luckily for all of us the Block Sister knew nothing of this. I had no problem after that getting the culprits to tidy their beds or fetch something from the kitchen or go and shave, etc. I have to confess that I took great pleasure in these small revenges. No one so much as *mentioned* spiders again.

With so many young men cooped up for months, even years, it was not surprising that some romances occurred with the nurses. This was frowned on because of the risk of infection, as well as propriety. But it happened, and they sometimes took the shape of hero (or heroine) worship.

Jasper

An earnest sergeant called Jasper seemed to admire me from a distance. Along with many others, he was up and about and almost ready to go home to his mother and sister. I found his devotion touching but embarrassing. I was also very worried that it was more than just the usual patient–nurse flirtation. He was not the sort to flirt. He was quiet and rather humble because he was 'only a sergeant', as he put it. Sure enough, the day he left, he asked me to go to tea with his family the following week. I was polite and firm in my refusal, but the entire family seemed to have come to take him home and added their entreaties. Without being very rude, I could do nothing but accept.

The afternoon was hugely difficult. Jasper's mother had baked cakes; an obviously new tablecloth was laid onto a small tea table in front of the fire. I was given the best armchair. His mother did not sit down at all, while his sister remained in the kitchen replenishing the teapot. He sat on the only other fireside chair, drinking cup after cup of tea, rather noisily, earning a reproving look from his mother.

I tried to talk about the hospital, as it was a common subject, but they all listened as if I were making a speech. After a while Jasper's mother asked about my family, so I told them about Robert and my parents.

The Country Nurse Remembers

Eventually, I felt that I could take my leave without appearing rude. To my consternation, Jasper was preparing to accompany me to the bus stop.

'I wanted them to see what a wonderful person you are,' he said on our way. 'Now they will see why I cannot possibly ask you to marry me.'

I held my breath. What on earth could I say?

He continued: 'You see, they knew that I loved you and have been pressing me to ask you to marry me. I knew it was not right. I'm only a sergeant, and I have no job now because of the TB. I live with my mother and sister in a council house. I am about twenty years older than you, and I have nothing to offer you. So I am saying "goodbye".'

He was staring across the street. He did not look at me once during this speech. I was so very sorry for him. He was a really decent person.

For once, I seemed to know how to deal with the situation.

'Thank you, Jasper, for telling me all this. You are a very nice person, and I am sure some girl will make you happy one day.'

He held onto the hand that I offered for a moment and then said, 'The bus is coming.'

I told Margaret all about it the next time we met. She listened with a surprised look. She had met Jasper. 'He is not right for you, I know, but it is a shame.' She paused and thought for a bit. Then she grinned. 'I suppose you could say that you have had a marriage *non*-proposal.'

I thought about Jasper for some time, and I decided that I must be a snob. I wouldn't want to live in the way that he did. I would be ashamed of being married to him. This was awful! *I* was awful! My family was nothing wonderful. We were very ordinary people, and yet I knew that I wanted something and someone with more education and more future than Jasper had. And yet he was so honest and had not tried to take advantage in any way, treating me with more respect than many well-educated men might.

Stupidly, I tried to talk to Mum and Dad about it.

'I don't know what you expect,' Mum said. 'He sounds a very nice person to me.'

Dad countered her by saying, 'He is far too old for you, and you don't want to marry beneath you.'

I should not have mentioned it!

Farewell to Ham Green

I enjoyed my six months at Ham Green. It was all so very different from the main hospitals: more relaxed, younger patients, and a lot of *fun*.

The young men, back from the most horrendous Japanese POW camps, never mentioned their ordeals, but I saw many signs of the brutality they had suffered: missing fingers, a missing ear in one case, scars from thrashings and deep marks from tight metal wrist restraints. If ever we approached them about these signs of their imprisonment, they would shrug them off with 'It doesn't hurt now!' or a jocular 'You should see the other guy!' They were all 'mates' and were determined to make up for lost time by having fun: childish, boyish fun for the most part, although there were times when we had to cast a blind eye on an empty bed late in the evening, knowing it would be filled by a very hung-over patient in the morning.

The village of Pill was reputed to have thirteen pubs! The lads had their own tankards, or beer glasses, that went to the pub with them. Although no one was likely to catch TB from a glass, the infection was not fully understood, and the boys were more readily accepted if complete with a glass of their own.

So they had fun. We young nurses were often chased around the wards (never again with a spider, though); the men would attack their mates' beds after we had gone and make them into the 'apple pie beds' of boarding schools, or they would pretend to be very ill by groaning horribly just to get a nurse to bend over them, only to grab her, pick her up and dump her on the bed or sit her on a high shelf.

Amazingly for an isolation hospital (or *any* hospital) there was a huge *wooden* sink in the block kitchen. It was very old and rough but still held water. It was not unusual for a couple of these young jokers to pick up a nurse and dump her in this sink, then turn the taps on. More than once I cycled back to the nurse's home wet through to change before Sister came round. None of us minded. These were young men who had suffered and witnessed terrible things, so we were happy to be part of their recovery—uncomfortable though it was sometimes!

The Old, Old Wards

On my return, reluctantly, to the Bristol hospitals, I found myself on night duty on a men's ward in the very oldest part of the oldest building. The hospital was built beside the docks and had suffered badly in the Blitz. Many advised knocking it down and rebuilding because it was very out of date, but there was not the money or the time to spare. We were still trying to catch up on the wartime backlog of patients—not just surgical cases, but the treatment of colitis, urinary problems, ulcers of various types, cancers (which were more frequently fatal then than they are now) and skin conditions.

I was now in my third year, having passed all the necessary exams along the way, so I was in charge of the ward at night. I had a junior, of course, and also an orderly, as there were many heavy, or old and rather confused, patients. An ex-RAMC man, he was not a dedicated nurse, feeling that the job was beneath him; he deeply resented having to take orders from a young nurse. He slept much of the night in one of the armchairs placed in the centre of the ward for 'up' patients and only worked in the morning or if I asked him to help me in the night.

There were two Night Sisters, who were always somewhere in the hospital for us to call on if there was some difficulty or emergency. When Sister's round was due, I always woke the orderly so that he would not be in trouble, but one night Sister was earlier than expected, and as we toured the ward I realised that he was sitting very obviously and comfortably right where we would pass.

We all had torches with rubber covers—so that we could see the patients without putting the lights on and could put the torch down without making a clatter. The sleeping orderly's bald head glowed in the light from Sister's torch. She stopped and gazed in disgust for a moment, then raised her rubber-covered torch and 'bopped'—the only word for it—his head. He leapt up with more oaths than Sister was prepared to put up with, and she ordered him off the ward immediately. She must have had him dismissed because no one saw him again; after that we shared a young, hard-working junior *male* nurse with another ward. Male nurses were very new, and he was the only one in the hospital.

One night, I was sitting alone at the desk with the light shining on my papers and across the polished wooden floor. Suddenly a movement caught my eye. I watched in horror as two enormous rats ran across the ward and disappeared into the sluices. What to do? I followed the intruders into the sluice, perhaps to shut them in, but they had found some way out, and there was no sign of them. I started thinking of bubonic plague (we were beside the docks) and Weil's disease (far more likely—the organisms are carried in the urine of rats, and, as rats have no bladder, they are dribbling urine constantly). I said nothing to my junior but called Sister from the ward office. She came at once, disinclined at first to believe me but soon convinced that I was not being hysterical. However, she felt that nothing could be done until the morning. Day Sister was appalled when I gave the report. Rats? In *her* ward?

The next night we were directed to a ward that had been speedily brought into use, as the other had been shut. It had been a children's fever ward before Ham Green had been built, and it was amusing to see the 'up' patients trying to sit in tiny chairs meant for five-year-olds.

God's Blessing

There had been an accident at the docks. The general hospital did not have a casualty department—that was at the Royal Infirmary—so I am not sure why we admitted two of the casualties. One man was only bruised and shocked, but the other one was carried in on a stretcher by very serious-looking ambulance men. (These were not the paramedics of today; the ambulance drivers were equipped with just first-aid knowledge.) It seemed that a large vessel had moved from its berth in an uncontrolled manner, causing 'domino effect' disasters along the quayside, with many injuries. The man was placed, still on the stretcher, on a bed. One of the ambulance men looked at me.

'He's conscious, but he has no pain. I can't understand it.'

The man was talking. I think I heard 'tell the wife' and 'poor Bert'. The doctor arrived and spoke reassuringly to him but looked shocked himself.

Only then did I get a look at the poor man.

I know many nurses in times of war, fire, terrorism and famine have seen and will continue to see and deal with all manner of horrors, but, although I had now seen death many times, it had been in controlled surroundings and was frequently not unexpected. This was quite different!

There seemed to be little recognisable shape to his body below the waist; his hands were badly crushed, but there was little bleeding. He lay quite still, conscious but unaware of his condition.

I began to try to undress him, but the fabric of his clothes seemed to be intertwined with his injured body. I looked at the doctor for guidance, but he merely shook his head.

I turned my attention to the man's boots. I untied the lace on one and began to remove it. As I picked up the boot, his foot came with it.

And still he was feeling nothing. 'Thank God for that' was my thought.

He died several hours later, still awake, still without pain, but also without the entire lower part of his body. The degree of shock had shut everything down, blood flow, pain, realisation: everything.

He had been working near the bollard that the huge steel hawser was wound around on the quayside. When the vessel pulled away from the side far too quickly, the hawser unwound out of control, whipping to and fro. Our poor man was caught in it and the lower half of his body torn apart.

Later in the little chapel, it seemed to me that although we knew the lack of pain was due to shock, it was also God's blessing.

The event was reported in the papers (without the horrendous details, of course), where our poor man was called 'Hawser Man'.

Time Rolls By

The years of training seemed to rush past in something of a blur. We were always busy at work, we went out in off-duty time if we had any money, we chatted in the nurses' home when we didn't and gradually I learnt more about everyday life, about the girls' families, about world affairs and about many things that girls of twelve or thirteen would already know these days.

For instance, I was well into my third year of training before I heard about lesbians—though I still thought that lesbians were just ladies living in the same house and being very fond of each other rather than wanting boyfriends. I think I was married and with a family before the details were made clear to me.

More amazing still was how the nurses' and doctors' remarks about the theatre porters went right over my head for nearly all my training. We had two hard-working, rather effeminate porters to take the patients to and from theatre. The good-natured teasing of some student doctors about 'all girls together' when they came into the anaesthetic room was a mystery to me. But I must have known somehow that it was a bit odd, because I did not feel I could ask about it. Today we would say that they were gay, but in those days that word only meant 'jolly' or 'happy'.

I was still an innocent and only gradually got to know things. I often wonder how many times I must have put my foot in it by saying the wrong thing! I think my father might have been slightly innocent in this way too, because I remember him remarking to me on one occasion, years later, that a certain woman was 'very masculine looking'. I don't think he had any idea that it was more than that.

My understanding of the patients, who came from varying backgrounds, went fairly smoothly. My association with all my colleagues, and those in authority over us, was sometimes smooth and sometimes very difficult. I didn't know when people were being serious or joking, for instance, and my own sense of humour was occasionally not understood by the other nurses. When I went out with a boy, I had little conversation and probably tried too hard to impress him. I felt inadequate *with* a boyfriend, but if I didn't have one I felt unwanted. The term 'boyfriend' in those days meant just that you were going out with a boy. We did a bit of kissing and cuddling at the end of an evening, usually on the steps of the nurses' home, with nurses passing in and out of the door all the time, but nothing more. The name implies much more now.

I was terrified of anyone in authority, and I am now sorry for many Sisters who tried to be if not friendly then at least chatty. I was totally unable to respond to their overtures. However, at the end of one three-month spell of night duty, which had been particularly arduous, the Night Sister (of whom *everyone* was afraid) came back to the ward specially in order to thank me for my hard work and to wish me luck for my future. My colleagues had difficulty believing me, but this incident taught me some self-esteem. Another boost came from a nurse who was leaving and wanted some help in composing her letter of resignation and her application for her next post. Several girls were there and offered all sorts of advice, to which she said: 'No, I want Julia to tell me what *she* thinks.' This small event helped me to see that I might have some aptitude outside hospital work and exams.

The Country Nurse Remembers

None of us were good 'citizens' because we were housed and fed and so had no worries about rent, food shopping, etc., and apart from clothes and fares our monthly salary was almost pocket money. That was the only budgeting we had to do. We led a hard-working and restricted life, but one that was also quite protected from outside responsibilities. So reaching out towards adulthood sometimes felt natural, but it often felt as though I were clawing my way over a precipice.

Gradually learning and gaining some authority of our own, we became second- and third-year nurses, and our salary rose to a dizzying £7 a month. After finals and before I left Bristol, I was 'Acting' Staff Nurse for a while. Prestige and responsibility, but no more money!

New young girls started their training, and I tried to remember how I had felt. I hope I was reasonably kind and understanding, but I'm sure my position of authority sometimes went to my head. But I noticed that from the start the new nurses all seemed to have far more confidence and an ease of manner that I was only then developing.

Finals loomed and off-duties were spent swotting, huddled under blankets in our rooms—there was no heating in the bedrooms, and the radio was always on in the warm sitting room.

There were practical exams in which I always felt frightened, but I must have passed because the results of both parts were satisfactory. There were also various subjects offered in which to gain prizes. I do not remember why I chose ophthalmology, but I was astounded when I won a prize. This was presented to me at the same time as the State Registration Certificate at a ceremony in the university. Sir Brian Horrocks, a wartime military hero, presented us all with whatever prize or certificate we had won and made a valiant attempt to talk to us: a lot of young girls! Having been used to hundreds of *men* under his command, he did not do a very good job, but we all laughed politely where we thought he was being funny. We couldn't wait for the tea afterwards, however.

Mum and Dad came, and I realised that it was the first time that they had ever seen me win anything, as parents had not been invited to school prize-givings.

I had made up my mind to leave and go to London to pursue my ambition to be a Theatre Nurse (or Sister one day), and this time Mum and Dad did not object, probably because I was now twenty-one, officially an adult and not a child just out of school. (Of my twenty-first birthday, I remember nothing at all.) Robert, too, now had his own friends at school, had joined the Cubs and was generally busy with his own affairs. I would miss him, though.

A State-Registered Nurse

Dad took me to the station in Bath.

I had saved a little money because my first post was not a live-in position and I would be paying rent for a small bedsit. I was nervous but excited to be starting at a prestigious and specialist hospital.

Dad stood on the platform as I waved from the train that bore me away to the next phase of my life.

I worked in the theatre of a large London hospital for a year until marrying, settling abroad and having a family. It would be twenty years before I once again resumed my career, when I became the District Nurse on a remote Scottish island.